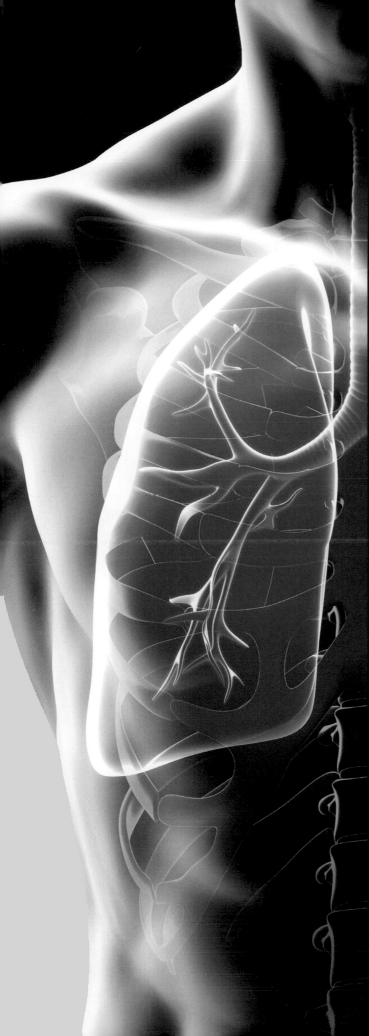

The Respiratory System
at a Glance

Fourth edition

Jeremy P.T. Ward PhD

Head of Department of Physiology
and Professor of Respiratory Cell Physiology
Division of Asthma, Allergy and Lung Biology
King's College London
London, UK

Jane Ward MBChB, PhD

Senior Lecturer
Department of Physiology
King's College London
London, UK

Richard M. Leach MD, FRCP

Consultant Physician and Honorary Senior
Lecturer
Guy's and St Thomas' Hospital Trust and
King's College London School of Medicine
St Thomas' Hospital
London, UK

WILEY Blackwell

Registered office: John Wiley & Sons, Ltd, The Atrium, Southern Gate, Chichester, West Sussex, PO19 8SQ, UK

Editorial offices: 9600 Garsington Road, Oxford, OX4 2DQ, UK
                      The Atrium, Southern Gate, Chichester, West Sussex, PO19 8SQ, UK
                      350 Main Street, Malden, MA 02148-5020, USA

For details of our global editorial offices, for customer services and for information about how to apply for permission to reuse the copyright material in this book please see our website at www.wiley.com/wiley-blackwell

Library of Congress Cataloging-in-Publication Data

Ward, Jeremy P. T., author.
  The respiratory system at a glance / Jeremy P.T. Ward, Jane Ward, Richard M. Leach. — Fourth edition.
       p. ; cm. — (At a glance series)
  Includes index.
  ISBN 978-1-118-76107-6 (pbk.)
  I. Ward, Jane, 1952– , author.   II. Leach, Richard M. (Haematologist), author.
III. Title.   IV. Series: At a glance series (Oxford, England)
  [DNLM: 1. Respiratory Physiological Phenomena.   2. Respiratory System – physiopathology.   3. Respiratory Tract Diseases. WF 102]
  RC731
  616.2—dc23

                                                          2015004640

A catalogue record for this book is available from the British Library.

Wiley also publishes its books in a variety of electronic formats. Some content that appears in print may not be available in electronic books.

Cover image: istock © Nerthuz

Set in Minion Pro 9.5/11.5 by Aptara
Printed and bound in Singapore by Markono Print Media Pte Ltd

3   2017

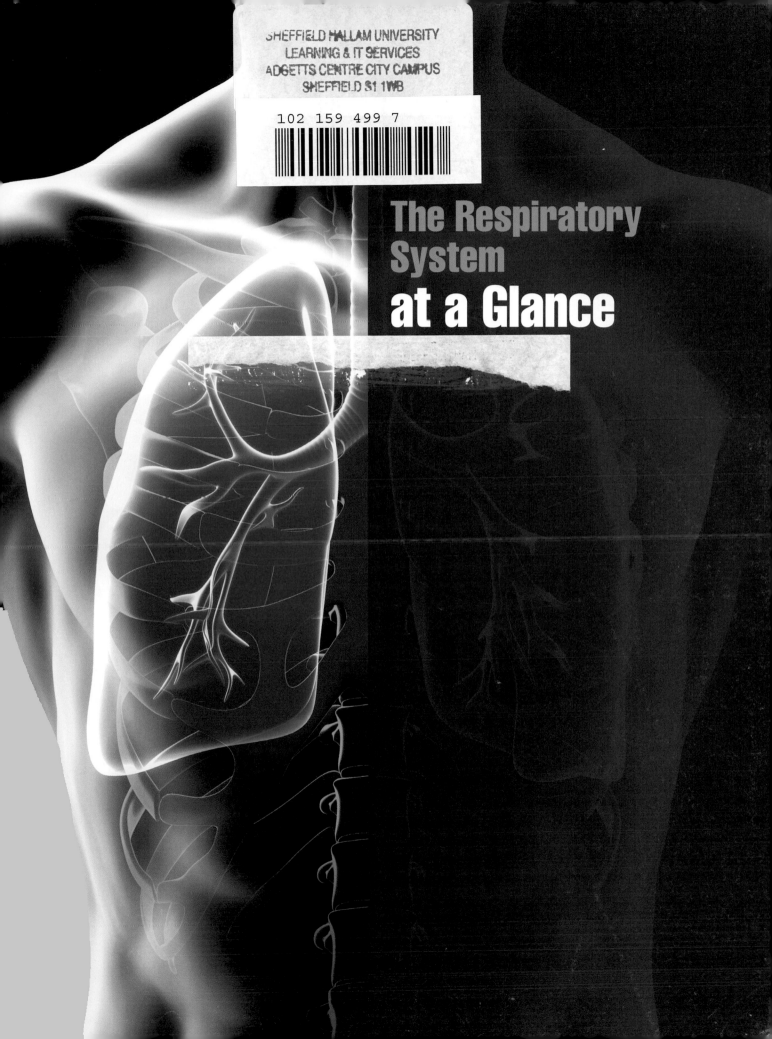

The Respiratory System
at a Glance

This title is also available as an e-book.
For more details, please see
www.wiley.com/buy/9781118761076
or scan this QR code:

Contents

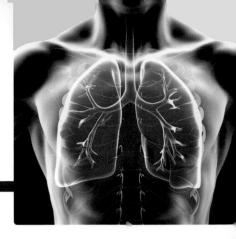

Preface to fourth edition

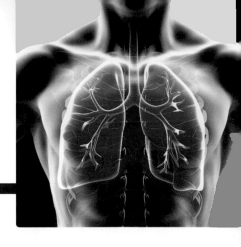

The medical curriculum is constantly being reviewed, but all modern curricula interleave basic and clinical science, physiology and pathophysiology. Clinical examples and cases provide relevance to and assist understanding of the underlying basic science, and basic science concepts help in the understanding of the pathophysiology and treatment of disease. *The Respiratory System at a Glance* is designed to support students following all programmes of study that integrate core aspects of basic science, pathophysiology and clinical medicine, including treatment. As such, it should be useful to medical students throughout their training, and also to other healthcare professions, including nursing.

As with other volumes in the *At a Glance* series, it is based around a two-page spread for each main topic, with figures and text complementing each other to give an overview at a glance. Case studies based on some of the most commonly encountered conditions are also provided on the companion website, and can be used for both basic science and clinical study. Although primarily designed for revision, the book covers all the core elements of the respiratory system and its major diseases, and as such could be used as a main text in the first couple of years of the course. It is advised, however, that additional reference to more detailed textbooks will aid deeper and wider understanding of the subject. This is particularly the case for the pathophysiological chapters, as a book this concise cannot hope to provide a complete guide to clinical practice.

In this fourth edition we have significantly revised the majority of chapters and improved or replaced figures to aid comprehension. In response to requests from readers, we now provide separate chapters on lung defence mechanisms and immunology, in keeping with their importance for most respiratory diseases, and there are now two chapters covering regulation of acid-base balance and acid-base disorders, an area that many find difficult. There are several additional case studies and self-assessment MCQs, now to be found on the companion website. We have hopefully corrected all errors in the last edition. We have been greatly assisted by our many colleagues and students who have kindly advised us and commented on the contents, but any errors and omissions are entirely our responsibility. We also thank the staff at Wiley, without whom we would not have been able to produce this edition.

Jeremy P.T. Ward
Jane Ward
Richard M. Leach

Acknowledgement

We would like to thank Charles M. Wiener, Professor of Medicine and Physiology at John Hopkins School of Medicine, Baltimore, USA, for his contribution to the original concept and the first and second editions of this book.

Units and symbols

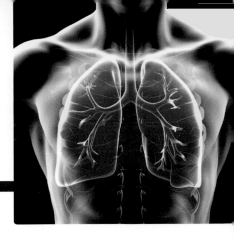

Units

The medical profession and scientific community generally use SI (Systéme International) units.

Pressure conversion: SI unit of pressure: 1 pascal (Pa) = 1 N/m^2. As this is small, in medicine the kPa (=10^3 Pa) is more commonly used. Note that millimetres of mercury (mmHg) are still the most common unit for expressing arterial and venous blood pressures, and low pressures - e.g. central venous pressure and intrapleural pressure - are sometimes expressed as centimetres of H_2O (cmH_2O). Blood gas partial pressures are reported by some laboratories in kPa and by some in mmHg, so you need to be familiar with both systems.

1 kPa = 7.5 mmHg = 10.2 cmH_2O
1 mmHg = 1 torr = 0.133 kPa = 1.36 cmH_2O
1 cmH_2O = 0.098 kPa = 0.74 mmHg
1 standard atmosphere ($\approx$1 bar) = 101.3 kPa = 760 mmHg =1033 cmH_2O

Contents are often expressed per 100 mL (dL), and these need to be multiplied by 10 to give the standard SI unit per litre. Contents are also increasingly being expressed as mmol/L. For haemoglobin: 1 g/dL = 10 g/L = 0.062 mmol/L. For ideal gases (including oxygen and nitrogen): 1 mmol = 22.4 mL standard temperature and pressure dry (STPD; see Chapter 4). For non-ideal gases, such as nitrous oxide and carbon dioxide: 1 mmol = 22.25 mL STPD. Technically, concentrations of ions in solution (e.g. [H$^+$], [K$^+$]) should be expressed as mole equivalents (e.g. mEq), but as there is no difference either numerically or in meaning we have mostly followed the convention of using molar concentrations.

Standard symbols

Primary symbols

F = Fractional concentration of gas
C = Content of a gas in blood
V = Volume of a gas
P = Pressure of partial pressure
S = Saturation of haemoglobin with oxygen
Q = Volume of blood

A dot over a letter means a time derivative, e.g. $\dot{V}$ = ventilation (L/min); $\dot{Q}$ = blood flow (L/min)

Secondary symbols

Gas: I = Inspired gas
E – Expired gas
A = Alveolar gas
D = Dead-space gas
T = Tidal
B = Barometric
ET = End-tidal

Blood: a = Arterial
v = Venous
c = Capillary
A dash means mixed or mean
e.g. $\bar{v}$ = Mixed venous
A′ after a symbol means end
e.g. c′ = End-capillary

Tertiary symbols

O_2 = Oxygen
CO_2 = Carbon dioxide
CO = Carbon monoxide

Examples

$\dot{V}O_2$ = Oxygen consumption
$P_A co_2$ = Alveolar partial pressure of carbon dioxide

Typical values

Typical inspired, alveolar and blood gas values in healthy young adults are shown in the table below. Ranges are given for arterial blood gas values. Mean arterial P_{O_2} falls with age, and by 60 years is about 11 kPa/82 mmHg. Typical values for lung volumes and other lung function tests are given in the appropriate chapters. Ranges for many values are affected by age, sex and height, as well as by the method of measurement, and hence it is necessary to refer to appropriate nomograms.

Inspired P_{O_2} (dry, sea level)	21 kPa	159 mmHg
Alveolar P_{O_2}	13.3 kPa	100 mmHg
Arterial P_{O_2}	12.5 (11.2–13.9) kPa	94 (84–104) mmHg
A–a P_{O_2} gradient	<2 kPa	<15 mmHg (greater in elderly)
Arterial oxygen saturation	>97%	
Arterial oxygen content	200 mL/L	20 mL/dL
Inspired P_{CO_2}	0.03 kPa	0.2 mmHg
Alveolar P_{CO_2}	5.3 (4.7–6.1) kPa	40 (35–45) mmHg
Arterial P_{CO_2}	5.3 (4.7–6.1) kPa	40 (35–45) mmHg
Arterial CO_2 content	480 mL/L	48 mL/dL
Arterial $[H^+]$/pH	35–45 nmol/L	7.45–7.35
Resting mixed venous P_{O_2}	5.3 kPa	40 mmHg
Resting mixed venous O_2 content	150 mL/L	15 mL/dL
Resting mixed venous O_2 saturation	75%	
Resting mixed venous P_{CO_2}	6.1 kPa	46 mmHg
Resting mixed venous CO_2 content	520 mL/L	52 mL/dL
Arterial $[HCO_3^-]$	24 (21–27) mmol/L	

List of abbreviations

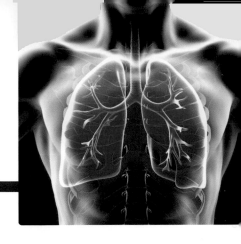

A–a gradient   (A-a P_{O_2}) gradient, the difference between ideal alveolar and arterial P_{O_2}

AAT α_1-antitrypsin

AHI   apnoea plus hypopnoea index

AIDS   acquired immune deficiency syndrome

AIP   acute interstitial pneumonia/pneumonitis (Hamman-Rich syndrome)

ALI   acute lung injury

ANA   anti-nuclear antibody

ANCA   anti-neutrophil cytoplasmic antibody

AP   anterior-posterior

ARDS   acute (formerly adult) respiratory distress syndrome

ATPS   ambient temperature and pressure saturated

ATS   American Thoracic Society (guidelines)

BAL   bronchoalveolar lavage

BALT   bronchus-associated lymphoid tissue

BCG   bacille Calmette-Guérin

BiPAP   bilevel positive airway pressure, biphasic positive airway pressure

BP   blood pressure

BTPS   body temperature and pressure saturated

BTS   British Thoracic Society (guidelines)

CA   carbonic anhydrase

cAMP   cyclic adenosine monophosphate

CAP   community-acquired pneumonia

CCF   congestive cardiac failure

CF   cystic fibrosis

CFA   cryptogenic fibrosing alveolitis

CFTR   cystic fibrosis transmembrane conductance regulator

C_L   lung compliance = $\Delta V/\Delta P$, where P = alveolar – intrapleural pressure

CMV   controlled mechanical ventilation

CMV   cytomegalovirus

CNS   central nervous system

COAD   chronic obstructive airway disease (synonymous with COPD, COLD)

COLD   chronic obstructive lung disease (synonymous with COAD, COPD)

COPD   chronic obstructive pulmonary disease (synonymous with COAD, COLD)

COX   cyclooxygenase

CPAP   continuous positive airway pressure

CREST   calcinosis, Raynaud's phenomenon, esophageal involvement, sclerodactyly and telangiectasia

CSA   central sleep apnoea

CSF   cerebrospinal fluid

CT   computed tomography

CTPA   computed tomography pulmonary angiogram

CWP   coal worker's pneumoconiosis

CXR   chest X-ray

DIP   desquamative interstitial pneumonia

$D_L{co}$ diffusing capacity of the lungs for carbon monoxide

$D_L g$ diffusing capacity of the lungs for gas

$D_L O_2$ diffusing capacity of the lungs for oxygen

DRG   dorsal respiratory group

DVT   deep venous thrombosis

EBV   Epstein–Barr virus

ECG   electrocardiogram

ECMO   extracorporeal membrane oxygenation

ECP   eosinophil cationic protein

EEG   electroencephalogram

EGF   epidermal growth factor

ELISA   enzyme-linked immunoassay

EMG   electromyogram

EOG   electrooculogram

ERV   expiratory reserve volume

ESR   erythrocyte sedimentation rate

FDG   fluorodeoxyglucose

FDG PET   fluorodeoxyglucose positron emission tomography

FEF_{25-75}   mean forced expiratory flow over middle 50% of forced vital capacity

FER   forced expiratory ratio

FEV_1   forced expiratory volume in 1 second

FEV_1/FVC FEV_1 expressed as a fraction, or more usually a percentage of FVC (= FER)

FGF   fibroblast growth factor

FRC   functional residual capacity

FVC   forced vital capacity

GBM   glomerular basement membrane

GM-CSF   granulocyte macrophage colony-stimulating factor

GU   genitourinary

HAART   highly active antiretroviral therapy

HAP   hospital acquired pneumonia

HCAP   healthcare-associated pneumonia

HIV   human immunodeficiency virus

HR   heart rate

HRCT	high-resolution computed tomography		**PEFR**	peak expiratory flow rate
ICU	intensive care unit		**PET**	positron emission tomography
IFN-γ	interferon-γ		**Pg**	prostaglandin, e.g. PgD_2
Ig	immunoglobulin, e.g. IgA, IgE, IgG and IgM		**PH**	pulmonary hypertension
IL	interleukin, e.g. IL-10		**pHa**	arterial pH
ILD	interstitial lung disease		**pK_A**	log of dissociation constant K_A
INPV	intermittent negative pressure ventilation		**PMF**	progressive massive fibrosis
IPF	idiopathic pulmonary fibrosis (synonymous with CFA)		**PMI**	point of maximal impulse (also known as Apex beat)
IPPV	intermittent positive pressure breathing		**PPD**	purified protein derivative
IRV	inspiratory reserve volume		**PPHN**	persistent pulmonary hypertension of the newborn
IVC	inferior vena cava		**PSP**	primary spontaneous pneumothorax
JVP	jugular venous pressure		**R**	respiratory gas exchange ratio
KCO	$D_L$co divided by alveolar volume or Krough coefficient		**RAD**	right axis deviation (electrocardiography)
KS	Kaposi's sarcoma		**RANTES**	regulated on activation normal T cell expressed and secreted
LA	left atrium, left atrial		**RAW**	airway resistance (mouth–alveolar pressure/airflow)
LDH	lactate dehydrogenase		**RBBB**	right bundle-branch block
LG	lymphomatoid granulomatosis		**RBC**	red blood cell
LIP	lymphocytic interstitial pneumonia		**REM**	rapid eye movement
LMWH	low-molecular-weight heparin		**RV**	residual volume
LT	leukotriene, e.g. LTC_4		**RV**	right ventricle
LV	left ventricle, left ventricular		**RVD**	restrictive ventilatory defect
MBP	major basic protein		**S_aO_2**	oxygen saturation of arterial blood (%)
MDR	multidrug resistant		**SC**	small cell
MI	myocardial infarction		**SCUBA**	self-contained underwater breathing apparatus
MIE	meconium ileus equivalent		**SIADH**	syndrome of inappropriate secretion of antidiuretic hormone
MMV	mandatory minute ventilation			
MOF	multiorgan failure		**SIMV**	synchronized intermittent mandatory ventilation
MRSA	methicillin-resistant *Staphylococcus aureus*			
MVV	maximal voluntary ventilation		**SLE**	systemic lupus erythematosus
NANC	non-adrenergic, non-cholinergic (nerves)		**SO_2**	oxygen saturation (oxygen content/oxygen capacity)
NHL	non-Hodgkin's lymphoma			
NIPPV	non-invasive positive pressure ventilation		**SP**	surfactant protein, e.g. SP-A
NRDS	neonatal respiratory distress syndrome		**STPD**	standard temperature and pressure dry
NREM	non-rapid eye movement		**SVC**	superior vena cava
NSAID	non-steroidal anti-inflammatory drug		**TB**	tuberculosis
NSC	non-small cell		**TGFβ**	transforming growth factor β
NSIP	non-specific interstitial pneumonia		**TLC**	total lung capacity
OSA	obstructive sleep apnoea		**T_LCO**	carbon monoxide transfer factor (alternative name for $D_L$co)
P_{50}	partial pressure at which haemoglobin is 50% saturated with O_2			
			UFH	unfractionated heparin
P_A	alveolar pressure		**UIP**	usual interstitial pneumonia
PA	posterior–anterior		**VAP**	ventilator-associated pneumonia
PA	pulmonary arterial		**V_A/Q**	ventilation–perfusion ratio (alveolar ventilation/blood flow in a lung region)
P_ACO	partial pressure of carbon monoxide in the alveoli			
			VC	vital capacity
P_aCO_2	arterial partial pressure of carbon dioxide		**VEGF**	vascular endothelial growth factor
P_ACO_2	alveolar partial pressure of CO_2		**VIP**	vasoactive intestinal peptide
PA F	platelet-activating factor		**$\dot{V}O_2$ max**	maximum oxygen consumption
PAH	pulmonary arterial hypertension		**VRG**	ventral respiratory groups
P_aO_2	partial pressure of oxygen in the arterial blood		**V_T**	tidal volume
			WBC	white blood cell
PCP	*Pneumocystis carinii* pneumonia		**WCC**	white cell count
$PD_{20}FEV_1$	provocative dose (e.g. of histamine or methacholine) that induces a 20% fall in FEV_1		**WG**	Wegener's granulomatosis
PDGF	platelet-derived growth factor			
PE	pulmonary embolus, pulmonary embolism			
PEEP	positive end-expiratory pressure			

About the companion website

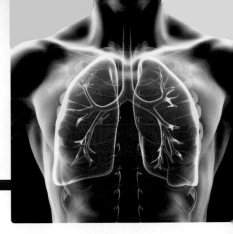

Don't forget to visit the companion website for this book:

www.wiley.com/go/ward/the respiratory system

There you will find valuable material designed to enhance your learning, including:

- Interactive multiple choice questions
- Case studies

Scan this QR code to visit the companion website:

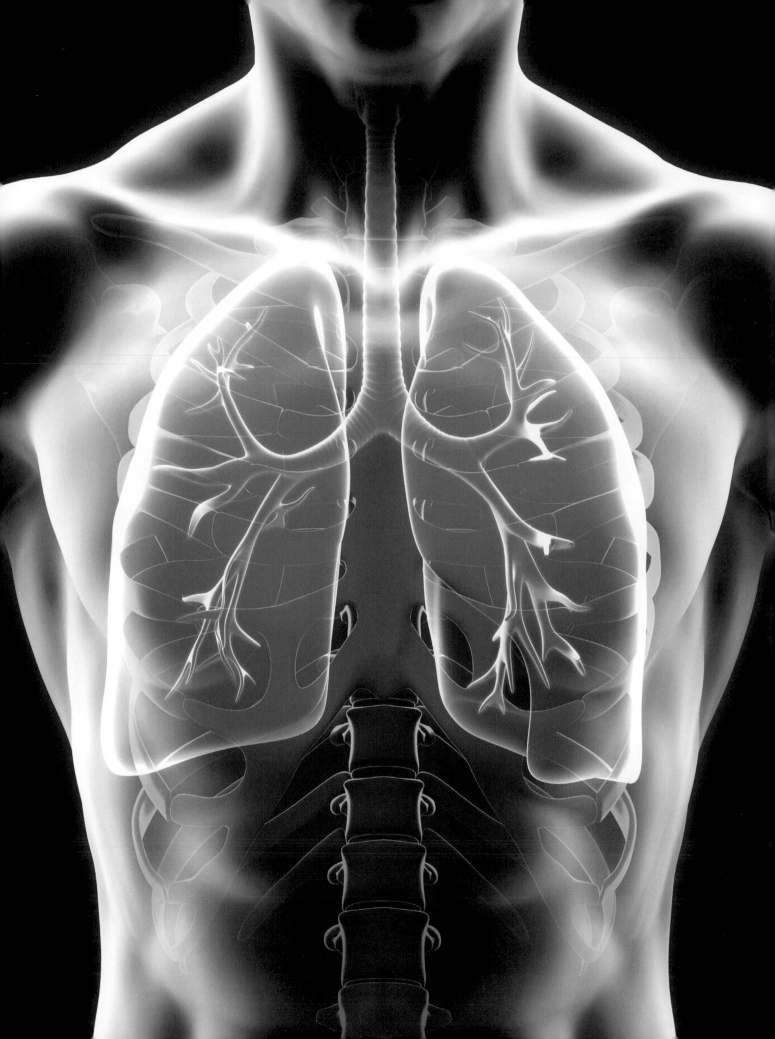

Structure and function

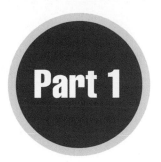

Part 1

Chapters

Structure of the respiratory system: lungs, airways and dead space

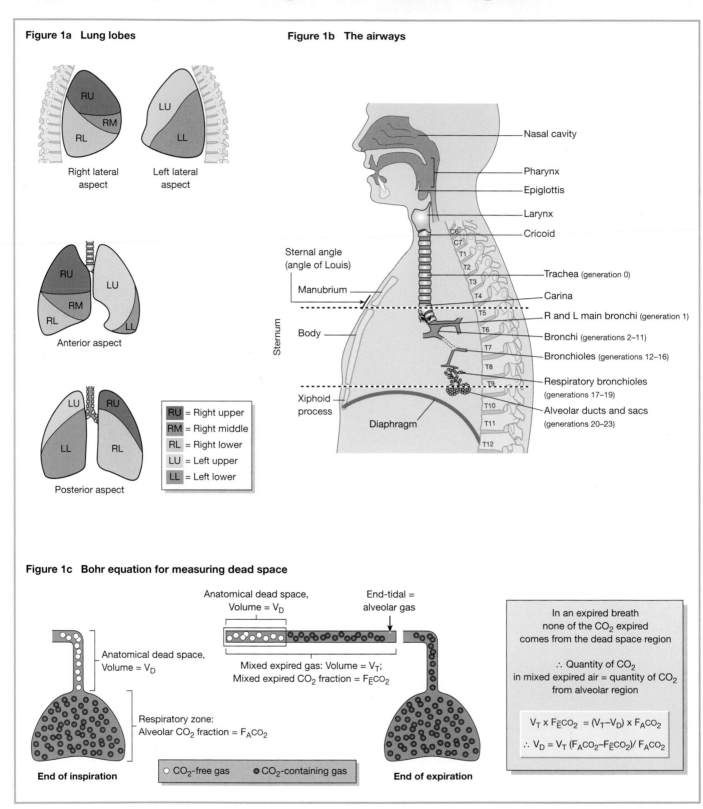

Figure 1a Lung lobes

Right lateral aspect

Left lateral aspect

Anterior aspect

Posterior aspect

RU = Right upper
RM = Right middle
RL = Right lower
LU = Left upper
LL = Left lower

Figure 1b The airways

Nasal cavity
Pharynx
Epiglottis
Larynx
Cricoid

Sternal angle (angle of Louis)
Manubrium
Sternum
Body

Trachea (generation 0)
Carina
R and L main bronchi (generation 1)
Bronchi (generations 2–11)
Bronchioles (generations 12–16)
Respiratory bronchioles (generations 17–19)
Alveolar ducts and sacs (generations 20–23)

Xiphoid process
Diaphragm

Figure 1c Bohr equation for measuring dead space

Anatomical dead space, Volume = V_D

End-tidal = alveolar gas

Anatomical dead space, Volume = V_D

Mixed expired gas: Volume = V_T;
Mixed expired CO_2 fraction = $F_{\bar{E}}CO_2$

Respiratory zone:
Alveolar CO_2 fraction = F_ACO_2

End of inspiration

○ CO_2-free gas   ● CO_2-containing gas

End of expiration

In an expired breath none of the CO_2 expired comes from the dead space region

∴ Quantity of CO_2 in mixed expired air = quantity of CO_2 from alveolar region

$$V_T \times F_{\bar{E}}CO_2 = (V_T - V_D) \times F_ACO_2$$

$$\therefore V_D = V_T (F_ACO_2 - F_{\bar{E}}CO_2) / F_ACO_2$$

The Respiratory System at a Glance, Fourth Edition. Jeremy P.T. Ward. © Jeremy P.T. Ward. Published 2015 by John Wiley & Sons, Ltd.

Lungs

The respiratory system consists of a pair of **lungs** within the **thoracic cage** (Chapter 2). Its main function is gas exchange, but other roles include speech, filtration of microthrombi arriving from systemic veins and metabolic activities such as conversion of angiotensin I to angiotensin II and removal or deactivation of serotonin, bradykinin, norepinephrine, acetylcholine and drugs such as propranolol and chlorpromazine. The **right lung** is divided by **transverse** and **oblique fissures** into three lobes: upper, middle and lower. The **left lung** has an **oblique fissure** and two lobes (Fig. 1a). Vessels, nerves and lymphatics enter the lungs on their medial surfaces at the lung root or **hilum**. Each lobe is divided into a number of wedge-shaped **bronchopulmonary segments** with their apices at the hilum and bases at the lung surface. Each bronchopulmonary segment is supplied by its own segmental bronchus, artery and vein and can be removed surgically with little bleeding or air leakage from the remaining lung.

The **pulmonary nerve plexus** lies behind each hilum, receiving fibres from both **vagi** and the second to fourth thoracic **ganglia** of the **sympathetic trunk**. Each vagus contains sensory afferents from lungs and airways, parasympathetic bronchoconstrictor and secretomotor efferents, and non-adrenergic, non-cholinergic (NANC). Sympathetic noradrenergic fibres supplying airway smooth muscle are sparse in humans, and the β_2-adrenergic receptors are stimulated by circulating catecholamines from the adrenal glands (Chapter 7).

Each lung is lined by a thin membrane, the **visceral pleura**, which is continuous with the **parietal pleura**, lining the chest wall, diaphragm, pericardium and mediastinum. The space between the parietal and visceral layers is tiny in health and lubricated with pleural fluid. The right and left pleural cavities are separate and each extends as the **costodiaphragmatic recess** below the lungs even during full inspiration. The parietal pleura is segmentally innervated by **intercostal nerves** and by the **phrenic nerve**, and so pain from pleural inflammation (**pleurisy**) is often referred to the chest wall or shoulder tip. The visceral pleura lacks sensory innervation.

Lymph channels are absent in alveolar walls, but accompany small blood vessels conveying lymph towards the hilar **bronchopulmonary nodes** and from there to **tracheobronchial nodes** at the tracheal bifurcation. Some lymph from the lower lobe drains to the **posterior mediastinal nodes**.

The **upper respiratory tract** consists of the nose, pharynx and larynx. The **lower respiratory tract** (Fig. 1b) starts with the trachea at the lower border of the **cricoid cartilage**, level with the sixth cervical vertebra (C6). It bifurcates into **right** and **left main bronchi** at the level of the **sternal angle** and T4/5 (lower when upright and in inspiration). The right main bronchus is wider, shorter and more vertical than the left, so inhaled foreign bodies enter it more easily.

Airways

The airways divide repeatedly, with each successive **generation** approximately doubling in number. The **trachea** and **main bronchi** have U-shaped cartilage, linked posteriorly by smooth muscle. Lobar bronchi supply the three right and two left lung lobes and divide to give **segmental bronchi** (generations 3 and 4). The total cross-sectional area of each generation is minimum here, after which it rises rapidly, as increased numbers more than make up for their reduced size. Generations 5–11 are small bronchi, the smallest being 1 mm in diameter. The lobar, segmental and small bronchi are supported by irregular plates of cartilage, with bronchial smooth muscle forming helical bands. **Bronchioles** start at about generation 12 and from this point onwards cartilage is absent. These airways are embedded in lung tissue, which holds them open like tent guy ropes. The **terminal bronchioles** (generation 16) lead to **respiratory bronchioles**, the first generation to have alveoli (Chapter 5) in their walls. These lead to **alveolar ducts** and **alveolar sacs** (generation 23), whose walls are entirely composed of **alveoli**.

The bronchi and airways down to the terminal bronchioles receive nutrition from the **bronchial arteries** arising from the descending aorta. The respiratory bronchioles, alveolar ducts and sacs are supplied by the **pulmonary circulation** (Chapter 14).

The airways from trachea to respiratory bronchioles are lined with **ciliated columnar or cuboidal epithelial cells**. Goblet cells and **submucosal glands** secrete **mucus**. Synchronous beating of cilia moves the mucus and associated debris to the mouth (**mucociliary clearance**) (Chapter 19). Epithelial cells forming the walls of alveoli and alveolar ducts are unciliated, and largely very thin **type I alveolar pneumocytes** (alveolar cells, *squamous epithelium)*. These form the gas exchange surface with the capillary endothelium (**alveolar–capillary membrane**). The **type II pneumocytes** make up only a small proportion of the alveolar surface area and are mostly found at the junction between alveoli. They are stem cells, which can divide following lung damage. They secrete **surfactant**, which reduces surface tension and has a role in lung immunity (Chapters 6 and 19). A similar substance is produced by the non-ciliated **Clara cells** found in the bronchiolar epithelium close to their junction with alveoli.

Dead space

The upper respiratory tract and airways as far as the terminal bronchioles do not take part in gas exchange. These **conducting airways** form the **anatomical dead space** whose volume (V_D) is normally about 150 mL. These airways have an air-conditioning function, warming, filtering and humidifying inspired air.

Alveoli that have lost their blood supply (e.g. because of a **pulmonary embolus**) no longer take part in gas exchange and form **alveolar dead space**. The sum of the anatomical and alveolar dead space is known as the **physiological dead space**, ventilation of which is wasted in terms of gas exchange. In health, all alveoli take part in gas exchange, so physiological dead space normally equals anatomical dead space.

The volume of a breath or **tidal volume** (V_T) is about 500 mL at rest. Resting **respiratory frequency** (f) is about 15 breaths/min, so the volume entering the lungs each minute, the **minute ventilation** ($\dot{V}$), is about 7500 mL/min (= 500×15) at rest. **Alveolar ventilation** ($\dot{V}_A$) is the volume taking part in gas exchange each minute. At rest, with a dead-space volume of 150 mL, alveolar ventilation is about 5250 mL/min (= $(500 - 150) \times 15$).

The **Bohr method** for measuring anatomical dead space is based on the principle that the degree to which dead-space gas (0% CO_2) dilutes alveolar gas (~5% CO_2) to give mixed expired gas (~3.5%) depends on its volume (Fig. 1c). **Alveolar gas** can be sampled at the end of the breath as **end-tidal gas**. The Bohr equation can be modified to measure physiological dead space by using arterial P_{CO_2} to estimate the CO_2 in the gas-exchanging or **ideal alveoli**.

The thoracic cage and respiratory muscles

Figure 2a The sternum and ribs and their relationship to the lungs and pleural cavities

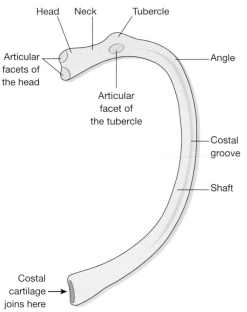

T1

Clavicle

Manubrium
Body } Sternum
Xiphoid process

Cardiac notch

Oblique fissure

Horizontal fissure

2
3
4
5
6
7
8
9
10

Oblique fissure

Costodiaphragmatic recess

Lung lobes

Pleural

Figure 2b Inferior aspect of a rib

Head   Neck   Tubercle

Articular facets of the head

Angle

Articular facet of the tubercle

Costal groove

Shaft

Costal cartilage joins here

Figure 2c An intercostal space

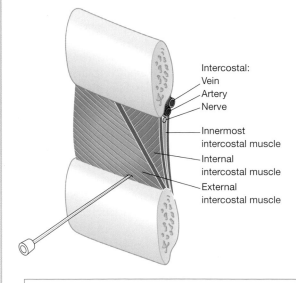

Intercostal:
Vein
Artery
Nerve

Innermost intercostal muscle

Internal intercostal muscle

External intercostal muscle

To avoid the neurovascular bundle, needles being passed through the intercostal space (e.g. to drain a pleural effusion) should pass close to the top of the rib

Figure 2d Inferior aspect of the diaphragm

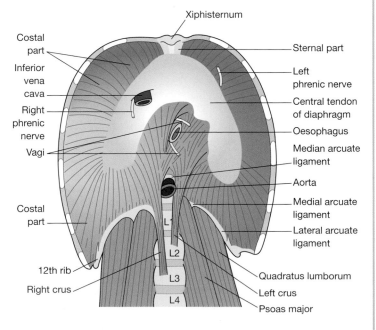

Xiphisternum

Costal part
Inferior vena cava
Right phrenic nerve
Vagi

Costal part

12th rib
Right crus

L1
L2
L3
L4

Sternal part
Left phrenic nerve
Central tendon of diaphragm
Oesophagus
Median arcuate ligament
Aorta
Medial arcuate ligament
Lateral arcuate ligament
Quadratus lumborum
Left crus
Psoas major

The Respiratory System at a Glance, Fourth Edition. Jeremy P.T. Ward. © Jeremy P.T. Ward. Published 2015 by John Wiley & Sons, Ltd.

Thoracic cage

The **thoracic cage** is composed of the **sternum, ribs, intercostal spaces** and **thoracic vertebral column**, with the **diaphragm** dividing the thorax from the abdomen.

The sternum

The dagger-shaped **sternum** has three parts. "The **manubrium**, with which the first and upper parts of the second costal cartilage and the clavicle articulate (Fig. 2a), lies at the level of the third and fourth thoracic vertebrae (see Fig. 2b)." The lower part of the second and the third to seventh ribs articulate with the **body of the sternum** (level with T5–T8). The angle between the manubrium and body at the cartilaginous **manubriosternal joint** forms the **sternal angle (angle of Louis)**, and this is a useful anatomical reference point. The small **xiphoid process** (xiphisternum) usually remains cartilaginous well into adult life.

The ribs and intercostal space

The first 7 (**true** or **vertebrosternal**) of the 12 pairs of ribs are connected to the sternum by their costal cartilages. The hyaline cartilages of the 8th, 9th and 10th (false or **vertebrochondral**) ribs articulate with the cartilage above, and the 11th and 12th are free (**floating** or **vertebral ribs**). A typical rib (Fig. 2b) has a **head** with two **facets** that articulate with the corresponding intervertebral disc and the vertebra above. The rib also articulates at the **tubercle** with the transverse process of the corresponding vertebra. The two articular regions act like a hinge, forcing the rib to move through an axis passing through these areas. The flattened shaft of the rib is weakest at the **angle of the rib** and this is where it tends to fracture in an adult. The upper two ribs, protected by the clavicle and the two floating ribs, are least likely to fracture. There is a cervical rib attached to the transverse process of C7 in 0.5% of people, and the presence of this rib may cause paraesthesia or vascular problems, due to pressure on the brachial plexus or subclavian artery.

Intercostal spaces contain **external intercostal muscles** whose fibres mostly pass downwards and forwards between the ribs, **internal intercostal muscles** whose fibres mostly pass downwards and backwards and an incomplete **innermost intercostal layer** (Fig. 2c). They are innervated by **intercostal nerves**, which are the anterior primary rami of **thoracic nerves**. **Intercostal veins**, **arteries** and **nerves** lie in grooves on the undersurface of the corresponding rib, with the vein above, artery in the middle and nerve below.

The diaphragm

The dome-shaped **diaphragm** (Fig. 2d) separates the thorax and abdomen and consists of a muscular peripheral part and a **central tendon**, which is partly fused with the pericardium. The muscular diaphragm takes its origin from the vertebrae and arcuate ligaments, the rib cage and the sternum. The **right crus** arises from the upper three lumbar vertebrae and the **left crus** from the upper two lumbar vertebrae. Their fibrous medial borders form the **median arcuate ligament** over the front of the aorta. The **medial** and **lateral arcuate ligaments** are thickenings of the fascia overlying the **psoas major** and **quadratus lumborum**, respectively. The costal part of the diaphragm is attached to the inner aspects of the 7th to 12th ribs and costal cartilages.

The sternal part originates as two slips from the back of the xiphisternum. The **phrenic nerves (C3, 4, 5)** supply motor fibres to the whole diaphragm and sensory fibres to the central part; pain from irritation of the diaphragm is often referred to the corresponding dermatome for C4, the shoulder tip. The lower intercostal nerves supply sensory fibres to the peripheral diaphragm. The aorta, thoracic duct and azygos vein pass through the diaphragm at the aortic opening at the level of T12. The oesophagus, branches of the left gastric artery and vein and both vagi pass through the oesophageal opening at the level of T10, and the inferior vena cava and right phrenic nerve pass through an opening at the level of T8.

Muscles of respiration

All inspiratory muscles act to increase thoracic volume, causing intrapleural and alveolar pressure to fall to create an alveolar–mouth pressure gradient, drawing air into the lungs. The expanded chest wall and lungs will recoil by themselves and quiet breathing uses no expiratory muscles.

The main inspiratory muscle, the **diaphragm**, moves down when it contracts, by about 1.5 cm during quiet breathing and 6–7 cm during deep breathing. During quiet breathing, the first rib remains fairly still and the **intercostal muscles** elevate and evert the succeeding ribs. The intercostal muscles also stiffen the intercostal spaces preventing them from being sucked in during inspiration. The **scalene muscles**, which insert into the first two ribs, are also active in normal inspiration. Raising the sternal ends of the upper ribs moves the sternum forwards and up, increasing the anterior–posterior dimension of the chest (the 'pump-handle' action). Raising the lateral shafts of the sloping lower ribs widens the chest transversely (the 'bucket-handle' action).

In quiet breathing in adults, ventilation is largely diaphragmatic. As the diaphragm contracts, it squashes the abdominal contents and raises intra-abdominal pressure, pushing out the abdominal wall and lower ribs. Consequently, in normal breathing the chest wall and the abdominal wall move out together during inspiration. If the diaphragm is paralysed, increased chest volume is produced entirely by raising the ribs, and as intrathoracic pressure falls in inspiration, the flaccid diaphragm is sucked into the chest and the abdomen moves in. This out-of-phase movement of the chest and abdominal walls is known as **paradoxical breathing**. In a high cervical cord transection, all respiratory muscles are paralysed, but when the damage is below the phrenic nerve roots (C3, 4, 5) breathing continues via the diaphragm alone. In the newborn, ribs are horizontal, so rib movements cannot increase the volume of the chest and breathing is entirely by the up-and-down action of the diaphragm or so-called **abdominal breathing**. As the ribs become more oblique with increasing age, there is an increased contribution of **thoracic breathing**.

When ventilation or resistance to breathing is increased, **accessory inspiratory muscles** aid inspiration. These include the **scalene muscles**, **sternomastoids** and **serratus anterior**. If the arms are fixed by grasping the edge of a table, contraction of the **pectoralis major**, which normally adducts the arm, helps expand the chest. When ventilation exceeds about 40 L/min, there is activation of expiratory muscles, especially **abdominal muscles (rectus abdominis, external and internal oblique)**, which speeds up recoil of the diaphragm by raising intra-abdominal pressure.

Pressures and volumes during normal breathing

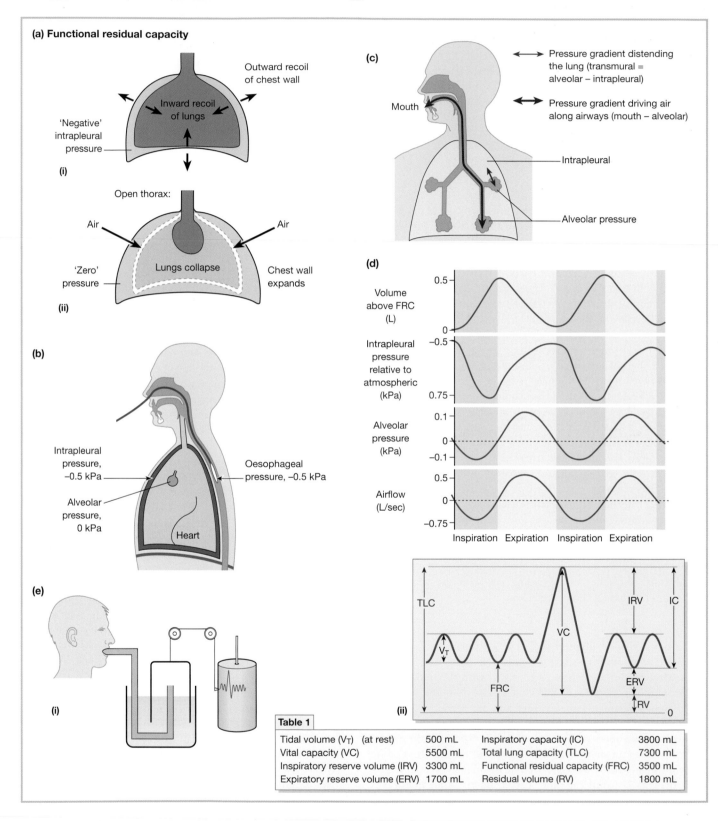

(a) Functional residual capacity

Outward recoil of chest wall

Inward recoil of lungs

'Negative' intrapleural pressure

(i)

Open thorax:

Air Air

'Zero' pressure

Lungs collapse

Chest wall expands

(ii)

(b)

Intrapleural pressure, −0.5 kPa

Oesophageal pressure, −0.5 kPa

Alveolar pressure, 0 kPa

Heart

(e)

(i)

(c)

Mouth

Pressure gradient distending the lung (transmural = alveolar − intrapleural)

Pressure gradient driving air along airways (mouth − alveolar)

Intrapleural

Alveolar pressure

(d)

Volume above FRC (L)

0.5

0

Intrapleural pressure relative to atmospheric (kPa)

−0.5

0.75

Alveolar pressure (kPa)

0.1

0

−0.1

Airflow (L/sec)

0.5

0

−0.75

Inspiration Expiration Inspiration Expiration

TLC

IRV IC

VC

V_T

FRC

ERV

RV

0

(ii)

Table 1

Tidal volume (V_T) (at rest)	500 mL		Inspiratory capacity (IC)	3800 mL
Vital capacity (VC)	5500 mL		Total lung capacity (TLC)	7300 mL
Inspiratory reserve volume (IRV)	3300 mL		Functional residual capacity (FRC)	3500 mL
Expiratory reserve volume (ERV)	1700 mL		Residual volume (RV)	1800 mL

The Respiratory System at a Glance, Fourth Edition. Jeremy P.T. Ward. © Jeremy P.T. Ward. Published 2015 by John Wiley & Sons, Ltd.

Functional residual capacity

The volume left in the lungs at the end of a normal breath is known as the **functional residual capacity (FRC)**. At FRC, the respiratory muscles are relaxed and its volume is determined by the elastic properties of the lungs and chest wall.

The natural resting volume of the lungs when removed from the body is very small and that of the chest wall, without the lungs, is about a litre larger than at FRC. In the living respiratory system, the lungs are sealed within the chest wall. Between these two elastic structures is the **intrapleural space**, which contains only a few millilitres of fluid. When the respiratory muscles are relaxed, the lungs and chest wall recoil in opposite directions, creating a subatmospheric ('negative') pressure in the space between them, and this tends to oppose the recoil of both the lungs and the chest wall. FRC occurs when the **outward recoil** of the chest wall exactly balances the **inward recoil** of the lungs (Fig. 3a). When the chest is opened, air enters the intrapleural space, the pressure becomes atmospheric and nothing opposes the recoil of the lungs and chest wall. The lungs shrink to a small volume and the chest wall springs out.

If the elastic recoil of either the lungs or the chest wall is abnormally large or small, FRC will be abnormal. In lung fibrosis, the lungs are stiff and have increased elastic recoil, so the balance point, and hence FRC, occurs at a small lung volume. In emphysema, there is loss of alveolar tissue and with it, loss of elastic recoil. When the respiratory muscles are relaxed, the reduced elastic recoil of the lungs offers less opposition to the outward recoil of the chest wall and FRC is increased (the **barrel chest** of emphysema). Increased FRC can also occur because of 'air trapping' (see Chapter 7).

Intrapleural pressure

The space between the **visceral pleura** lining the lungs and the **parietal pleura** lining the chest wall is so small that measuring **intrapleural pressure** with a needle risks puncturing the lung. Intrapleural pressure can be indirectly assessed from **oesophageal pressure** (Fig. 3b). The oesophagus is normally closed at the top and bottom except during swallowing and in the upright subject the oesophageal pressure is the same as in the neighbouring intrapleural space. The subject swallows either a miniaturized pressure transducer or a balloon containing a little air connected by a tube to an external manometer. Gravity affects the fluid-lined intrapleural space, and at FRC in an upright subject, the intrapleural pressure is about -0.5 kPa (-5 cmH$_2$O) at the apex of the lungs and about -0.2 kPa (-2 cmH$_2$O) at the bottom.

Pressures, flow and volume during a normal breathing cycle

During inspiration, the chest wall is expanded and intrapleural pressure falls (Fig. 3d). This increases the pressure gradient between the intrapleural space and alveoli (Fig. 3c), stretching the lungs. The alveoli expand and **alveolar pressure** falls, creating a pressure gradient between the mouth and alveoli,

causing air to flow into the lungs. The airflow profile closely follows that of alveolar pressure (Fig. 3d). During expiration, both intrapleural pressure and alveolar pressure rise. In quiet breathing, intrapleural pressure remains negative for the whole respiratory cycle, whereas alveolar pressure is negative during inspiration and positive during expiration. Alveolar pressure is always higher than intrapleural because of the recoil of the lung. It is zero at the end of both inspiration and expiration, and airflow ceases momentarily. When ventilation is increased, the changes of intrapleural and alveolar pressure are greater and in expiration intrapleural pressure may rise above atmospheric pressure. In forced expiration, coughing or sneezing, intrapleural pressure may rise to $+8$ kPa ($+60$ mmHg) or more.

Lung volumes

A **simple water-filled spirometer** (Fig. 3e(i)) trace best illustrates the important lung volumes. As the subject breathes in and out, the drum falls and rises and the pen, attached by a pulley system, produces a trace (Fig. 3e(ii)). Conventionally, volumes composed of two or more volumes are known as 'capacities', whereas those that cannot be subdivided are known as 'volumes'. The volume breathed in (or out) is known as the **tidal volume (V_T)**, and the trace shows several **resting tidal volumes**, which are typically about 500 mL. At the end of a normal quiet inspiration, the subject could breathe in more and this is the **inspiratory reserve volume (IRV)**. Similarly, the volume that he or she could exhale after a normal expiration is the **expiratory reserve volume (ERV)**. For the fourth breath, the subject breathes in and out as fully as possible. This maximum tidal volume is the **vital capacity (VC = V_T + IRV + ERV)**. At the end of a maximal breath out, the volume remaining in the lungs is the **residual volume**. FRC and **total lung capacity** are the volumes in the lungs at the end of a normal expiration and after a maximal breath in, respectively. Possible values for a man are given in Table 1. Although a zero volume line is shown (Fig. 3e(ii)), it is not possible to know where this actually is on a trace, because the subject cannot empty the lungs into the drum. For this reason, although illustrated in Fig. 3e(ii), volumes shown in red in Table 1 cannot be measured from a simple spirometer trace. They can be measured using **helium dilution** or **body plethysmography** (Chapter 22). The range of normal lung volumes is large and an individual's volumes must be assessed with the aid of **nomograms** that give the predicted value of each volume for the subject's age, sex and height.

Vital capacity during a forced expiration (FVC) and the volume exhaled in the first second (FEV$_1$) are important clinical measurements. Various types of spirometer have replaced the water-filled version for these measurements. These include the **bellows spirometer**, in which a stylus arm attached to the bellows scratches a trace onto waxed paper as the bellows fills with expired air and **electrospirometers**, which measure airflow and derive volumes by electrical integration. The volume against time spirograms produced with these spirometers are discussed in Chapter 22 and the flow against volume plots made possible by use of an electrospirometry are discussed in Chapter 7.

4 Gas laws

Figure 4a   Altitude, barometric pressure, O$_2$ fraction and PO$_2$

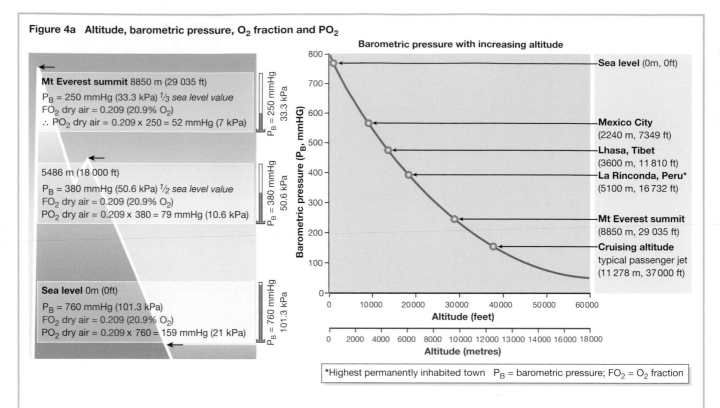

Mt Everest summit 8850 m (29 035 ft)

P_B = 250 mmHg (33.3 kPa) $^1/_3$ sea level value
FO$_2$ dry air = 0.209 (20.9% O$_2$)
∴ PO$_2$ dry air = 0.209 x 250 = 52 mmHg (7 kPa)

P_B = 250 mmHg
33.3 kPa

5486 m (18 000 ft)

P_B = 380 mmHg (50.6 kPa) $^1/_2$ sea level value
FO$_2$ dry air = 0.209 (20.9% O$_2$)
PO$_2$ dry air = 0.209 x 380 = 79 mmHg (10.6 kPa)

P_B = 380 mmHg
50.6 kPa

Sea level 0m (0ft)

P_B = 760 mmHg (101.3 kPa)
FO$_2$ dry air = 0.209 (20.9% O$_2$)
PO$_2$ dry air = 0.209 x 760 = 159 mmHg (21 kPa)

P_B = 760 mmHg
101.3 kPa

Barometric pressure with increasing altitude

Sea level (0m, 0ft)

Mexico City
(2240 m, 7349 ft)

Lhasa, Tibet
(3600 m, 11 810 ft)

La Rinconda, Peru*
(5100 m, 16 732 ft)

Mt Everest summit
(8850 m, 29 035 ft)

Cruising altitude
typical passenger jet
(11 278 m, 37 000 ft)

*Highest permanently inhabited town P_B = barometric pressure; FO$_2$ = O$_2$ fraction

Figure 4b   Correction factors for gas volumes

$$\text{Volume}_{(BTPS)} = \text{volume}_{(ATPS)} \left(\frac{273 + 37}{273 + t°C}\right)\left(\frac{P_B - P_{H_2O}}{P_B - 6.3^*}\right) \text{*47 if } P_B \text{ and } P_{H_2O} \text{ are in mmHg}$$

$$\text{Volume}_{(STPD)} = \text{volume}_{(ATPS)} \left(\frac{273}{273 + t°C}\right)\left(\frac{P_B - P_{H_2O}}{101^*}\right) \text{*760 if } P_B \text{ and } P_{H_2O} \text{ are in mmHg}$$

Figure 4c Partial pressure of a gas in a liquid

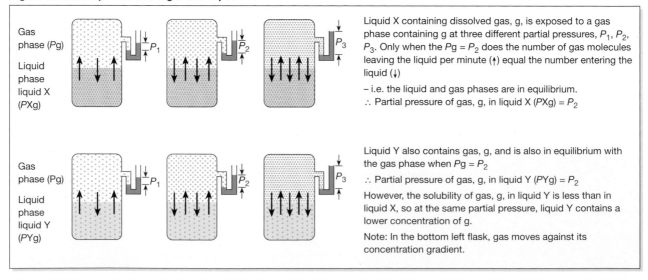

Gas phase (Pg)

Liquid phase liquid X (PXg)

Liquid X containing dissolved gas, g, is exposed to a gas phase containing g at three different partial pressures, P_1, P_2, P_3. Only when the $Pg = P_2$ does the number of gas molecules leaving the liquid per minute (↑) equal the number entering the liquid (↓)

– i.e. the liquid and gas phases are in equilibrium.

∴ Partial pressure of gas, g, in liquid X (PXg) = P_2

Gas phase (Pg)

Liquid phase liquid Y (PYg)

Liquid Y also contains gas, g, and is also in equilibrium with the gas phase when $Pg = P_2$

∴ Partial pressure of gas, g, in liquid Y (PYg) = P_2

However, the solubility of gas, g, in liquid Y is less than in liquid X, so at the same partial pressure, liquid Y contains a lower concentration of g.

Note: In the bottom left flask, gas moves against its concentration gradient.

The Respiratory System at a Glance, Fourth Edition. Jeremy P.T. Ward. © Jeremy P.T. Ward. Published 2015 by John Wiley & Sons, Ltd.

To understand the processes involved in respiration and how valid measurements are made, it is important to understand the behaviour of gases in both gas mixtures and liquids.

Fractional concentration and partial pressure of gases in a gas mixture

Dalton's law states that when two or more gases, which do not react chemically, are present in the same container, the total pressure is the sum of the partial pressures (the pressure that each gas would exert if isolated in the container).

The total pressure exerted by the atmosphere was traditionally measured by inverting a long mercury-filled glass tube over a mercury reservoir. At sea level, the height of the column supported is normally about 760 mm, so barometric pressure is 760 mmHg (1 mmHg $\cong$ 1 torr), which in SI units is about 101 kPa (1 kPa = 7.50 mmHg). Dried air contains approximately 21% oxygen (i.e. oxygen fraction (FO_2) $\approx$0.21). The remaining gases are nitrogen, 78.1%, and inert gases such as argon and helium, 0.9%, although for convenience these physiologically inert gases are often pooled as 'nitrogen, 79%'. Air is considered to be CO_2-free, as the amount present (0.04%) is very small. According to Dalton's law:

Dry partial pressure oxygen in inspired air (P_IO_2)

= oxygen fraction (FO_2) × total barometric pressure (P_B)

= $0.21 \times 101 (760) = 21.2$ kPa (159 mmHg)

At **altitude**, the oxygen fraction of air is unaltered, but barometric pressure is reduced, being about 33.3 kPa (250 mmHg) on the top of Everest (Fig. 4a).

Water vapour pressure

Air contains variable amounts of water vapour, depending on the water it has been exposed to and the temperature. The maximum or **saturated water vapour pressure** is higher in warm than in cool air: at 20°C, it is 2.33 kPa (17.5 mmHg), whereas at body temperature (37°C), it is 6.3 kPa (47 mmHg). The **relative humidity** (actual/saturated water vapour pressure × 100%) of inspired air varies with the weather; if it is 40% at 20°C, water vapour pressure will be 0.9 kPa (7 mmHg). The presence of water vapour means that ambient FO_2 and FN_2 are usually a little lower than the dry fractions given above. Air passing down the airways quickly reaches body temperature (37°C) and 100% saturation. Total pressure remains close to barometric, so the added water vapour causes significant dilution of the other gases. The available pressure for the other gases is therefore P_B – 6.3 kPa (P_B – 47 mmHg).

The **partial pressure of moist inspired oxygen (P_IO_2)** = 0.21 × (P_B – saturated vapour pressure at 37°C).

Moistened inspired P_IO_2 is always 1.3 kPa (= 0.21 × 6.3) or 10 mmHg less than dry PO_2. Note that this has a proportionally greater effect on P_IO_2 at high altitude than at sea level. If dry air is saturated with water at 37°C, at sea level P_IO_2 falls by 6% from 21.2 to 19.9 kPa (159–149 mmHg); on the summit of Everest, P_IO_2 falls from 7.0 to 5.7 kPa (52–42 mmHg), a 19% reduction.

The effect of pressure and temperature on gas volumes

The inverse relationship between the volume of a perfect gas and its pressure, described by **Boyle's law** (P $\propto$ 1/V), and the direct relationship between volume and absolute temperature (= 273 + °C), described by **Charles' law** (V $\propto$ T), are important when measuring gas volumes. Expired gas collected in a bag or spirometer will shrink, both because of the direct effect of falling temperature (Charles' law) and because water vapour condenses as temperature falls. To enable valid comparisons, volumes at **ambient temperature and pressure saturated with water (ATPS)** are corrected to those they would occupy under standard conditions. For measurements of lung volumes, this is for **body temperature and pressure saturated with water (BTPS)**. For O_2 consumption or CO_2 production, **standard temperature and pressure dry (STPD)** (0°C, 101.3 kPa (760 mmHg), $PH_2O = 0$) are usually used, so that each litre contains the same number of molecules (1 mole $\approx$ 22.4 L).

Boyle's law, Charles' law and the reduction of saturated vapour pressure with temperature are combined in the equations for correcting volumes given in Figure 4b.

Gases dissolved in liquids

If a liquid is exposed to a gas to which it does not react, gas particles will move into the liquid. **Henry's law** states that the number of molecules dissolving in the liquid is directly proportional to the partial pressure at the surface of the gas.

The constant of proportionality is the solubility of the gas in the liquid, and it is affected by the gas, the liquid and the temperature, tending to fall as temperature rises.

Content of dissolved gas X in a liquid Y = solubility of X in Y × partial pressure of X at surface

The **partial pressure of a gas in a liquid** or **gas tension** is a more difficult concept than that of partial pressure in a gas phase, where we can visualize the pressure of the molecules holding up a column of mercury. The molecules of the gas in the liquid phase will move about in the liquid and have a tendency to escape from the surface, which can be opposed by molecules of the same gas in a gas phase in contact with the liquid (Fig. 4c). If the partial pressure of the gas in the gas phase is altered until there is no net movement of gas between the gas phase and the liquid phase, the gas and liquid are said to be in equilibrium. By definition, the partial pressure of a gas in a liquid is equal to the partial pressure of that gas in a gas phase with which it is in equilibrium. Partial pressure gradient (not concentration gradient) always determines the direction of movement between phases such as a gas and a liquid phase.

Note on time-derivative symbols

Standard symbols used in respiratory physiology are given in Units and Symbols on page ix. Time derivatives are properly denoted by a dot over the symbol (e.g. $\dot{V}_A$, alveolar ventilation in L/min, see Units and Symbols on page ix). However, for terms such as the ventilation–perfusion ratio (VA/Q) the dots are often omitted, and this convention is followed throughout this book.

5 Diffusion

Figure 5a The alveolar–capillary membrane

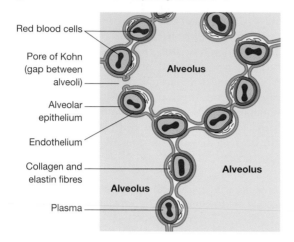

Red blood cells

Pore of Kohn
(gap between
alveoli)

Alveolus

Alveolar
epithelium

Endothelium

Collagen and
elastin fibres

Alveolus

Alveolus

Plasma

Figure 5b Transfer of gases across alveolar–capillary membrane

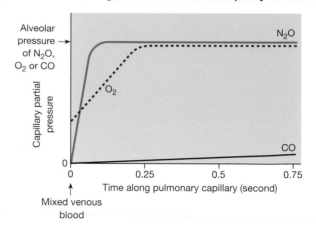

Alveolar
pressure →
of N$_2$O,
O$_2$ or CO

Capillary partial pressure

N$_2$O

O$_2$

0

CO

0   0.25   0.5   0.75

Time along pulmonary capillary (second)

↑
Mixed venous
blood

Figure 5c Diffusion through a sheet of tissue

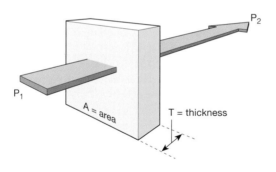

P$_2$

P$_1$

A = area

T = thickness

Figure 5d The oxygen cascade: oxygen tension from ambient air to mitochondria

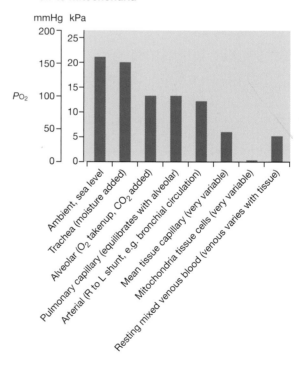

mmHg   kPa

Po$_2$

200 — 25
150 — 20
     15
100 — 10
 50 — 5
  0 — 0

Ambient, sea level
Trachea (moisture added)
Alveolar (O$_2$ takenup, CO$_2$ added)
Pulmonary capillary (equilibrates with alveolar)
Arterial (R to L shunt, e.g. bronchial circulation)
Mean tissue capillary (very variable)
Mitochondria tissue cells (very variable)
Resting mixed venous blood (venous varies with tissue)

Figure 5e The diffusion path through the alveolar–capillary membrane

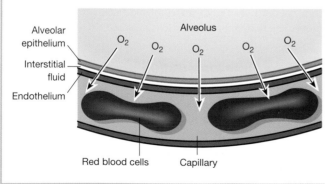

Alveolar
epithelium

Alveolus

O$_2$ O$_2$ O$_2$ O$_2$ O$_2$

Interstitial
fluid

Endothelium

Red blood cells   Capillary

The Respiratory System at a Glance, Fourth Edition. Jeremy P.T. Ward. © Jeremy P.T. Ward. Published 2015 by John Wiley & Sons, Ltd.

Oxygen and carbon dioxide are transported in the body by a mixture of **bulk flow** and **diffusion**. Bulk flow, generated by differences in total fluid pressure, is important in most of the airways and in transporting blood containing these gases between pulmonary and tissue capillaries. Diffusion, driven by partial pressure differences, is important in the last few millimetres of the airways, across the alveolar–capillary membrane and between tissue capillaries and mitochondria.

The alveolar–capillary membrane

Adult male lungs contain about 300 million alveoli, approximately 0.2 mm in diameter (Fig. 5a). Between neighbouring alveoli are two layers of **alveolar epithelium** each resting on a basement membrane, enclosing the interstitial space, containing **pulmonary capillaries**, elastin and **collagen fibres**. The **alveolar epithelium** and **capillary endothelium** form the **alveolar-capillary membrane**, through which gases diffuse. It is very thin (<0.4 μm), except where collagen and elastin fibres are concentrated, with a total surface area of about 85 m². There are two types of alveolar epithelial cells. **Type I pneumocytes** line the alveoli and are relatively devoid of organelles. The round **type II pneumocytes** have large nuclei, microvilli and contain striated osmiophilic lamellar bodies storing surfactant, an important component of alveolar lining fluid (Chapter 6).

Diffusion and perfusion limitation

If gas containing the poorly soluble gas nitrous oxide (N_2O) is inhaled, pulmonary capillary PN_2O rises and quickly equilibrates with alveolar PN_2O (Fig. 5b). With no alveolar–capillary partial pressure gradient remaining, diffusion ceases along the rest of the pulmonary capillary and uptake can only be increased by increasing pulmonary capillary blood flow. N_2O uptake is said to be **perfusion limited**. In contrast, when breathing a carbon monoxide (CO) containing mixture, the CO combines so avidly with haemoglobin that pulmonary capillary PCO rises little. The pressure gradient driving diffusion is preserved along the capillary, and CO uptake would not be increased by increased perfusion. Improved ease of diffusion, with reduced thickness or increased area of the alveolar–capillary membrane, would increase CO uptake. CO transfer is **diffusion limited**. Oxygen transfer lies between these two extremes, but is normally perfusion limited.

Factors affecting diffusion across a membrane (Fick's and Graham's laws)

For a sheet of tissue of area A and thickness T, through which gas g is passing driven by the pressure gradient, $P_1 - P_2$ (Fig. 5c):

$$\text{Rate of transfer of gas, } g \propto \frac{A}{T}(P_1 - P_2)$$

The constant of proportionality

$$= \frac{\text{Solubility of the gas in the membrane(s)}}{\sqrt{\text{Molecular weight of the gas}}}$$

Although the molecular weight of CO_2 is about 1.4 times that of O_2, it is about 20 times more soluble, and so diffuses more easily.

For the alveolar–capillary membrane, the pressure gradient driving diffusion is alveolar (P_A) minus mean pulmonary capillary ($P_{\bar{C}}$). The constants (s, mw, A and T) can be combined to give a single constant, the **diffusing capacity** (D_Lg) of the lungs for gas, g:

$$\text{Rate of transfer of gas, } g = D_Lg(P_A - P_{\bar{C}})$$

$$\text{Oxygen diffusing capacity, } D_LO_2$$

$$= \frac{\text{Oxygen uptake from the lungs }(\dot{V}O_2)}{P_AO_2 - P_{\bar{C}}O_2}$$

Although measurement of D_LO_2 is desirable, it is not possible because mean capillary PO_2 ($P_{\bar{C}}O_2$) cannot be measured. CO diffuses through the same pathway as O_2, and its rate of diffusion is affected by the same factors that affect oxygen transfer. However, unlike D_LO_2, D_LCO is measurable. Once CO arrives in the pulmonary capillary blood, it too combines with haemoglobin. Haemoglobin has approximately 240 times the affinity for CO than it does for O_2, and consequently as CO is transferred, almost all of it enters chemical combination and the mean pulmonary capillary PCO can be assumed to be zero. This simplifies the equation to:

$$D_LCO = \frac{\text{Carbon monoxide uptake from the lungs }(\dot{V}CO)}{P_ACO}$$

Several methods are used for measuring D_LCO, but all involve breathing a low level of CO (e.g. 0.3%). By sampling exhaled gas, CO uptake, mean alveolar PCO and therefore D_LCO can be calculated. The normal value depends on the method used, but is about 15–30 mL/min per mmHg (112–225 mL/min per kPa). A tracer gas, such as helium, is included in the gas mixture so that alveolar volume can also be measured (see Chapter 22). D_LCO is divided by alveolar volume to give an index (KCO) that corrects for different lung volumes. As both D_LO_2 and D_LCO are affected by the rate of gas combination with haemoglobin, in addition to factors affecting diffusion, the alternative term, transfer factor (T_LO_2 and T_LCO), is more commonly used in Europe.

Factors affecting D_LCO (T_LCO)

D_LCO is lowered by reduced alveolar–capillary membrane area in emphysema, pulmonary emboli or lung resection and by increased thickness in pulmonary oedema. In pulmonary fibrosis the alveolar–capillary membrane is both thickened and reduced in area, giving a low D_LCO with a low but less affected KCO. Increased pulmonary blood volume in exercise increases the effective area increasing D_LCO. D_LCO is increased with polycythaemia and reduced in anaemia. D_LCO is therefore non-specific, but it is sensitive and may reveal abnormalities when other lung function tests are normal. Hypoventilation does not affect D_LCO because the reduced CO uptake is caused by reduced P_ACO.

The oxygen cascade (Fig. 5e) shows how PO_2 falls between air and mitochondria. Mitochondrial oxidative phosphorylation will cease when PO_2 falls below 1 mmHg (0.13 kPa), and this ultimately limits the capillary PO_2 that can be tolerated and therefore the amount of oxygen that can be removed as blood passes through the tissues. Capillary PO_2 must remain high enough to drive diffusion to cells at a rate sufficient to match oxygen consumption and maintain mitochondrial PO_2 above this critical level. Although the fall in PO_2 at different stages of the oxygen transport system is often regarded as an unfortunate inefficiency, more recently it has been suggested that, in sea level dwellers, it helps protect cells from an excessively high PO_2, which can be toxic because of increased production of reactive oxygen species. However, the step falls in PO_2 are unhelpful at very high altitude, where the problem is keeping the tissue PO_2 high enough.

6 Lung mechanics: elastic forces

Figure 6a Static pressure–volume loop

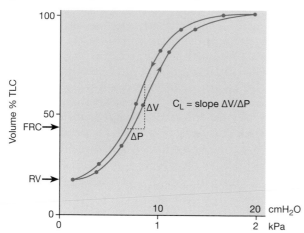

$$C_L = \text{slope } \Delta V / \Delta P$$

Transmural pressure (= – intrapleural pressure since measurements taken at zero airflow)

RV = Residual volume   FRC= Functional residual capacity
TLC= Total lung capacity C_L= Lung compliance

Figure 6b Dynamic pressure–volume loop

If intrapleural pressure and volume are recorded continuously (lower panel), a pressure–volume loop (upper panel) can be constructed from pairs of simultaneous measurements of volume, e.g. (b) with pressure (b'). Alternatively the pressure and volume signals can be fed into an X-Y plotter.

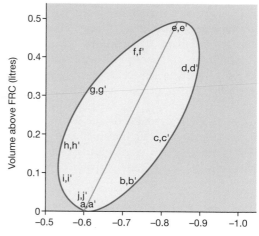

Intrapleural pressure relative to atmospheric (kPa)

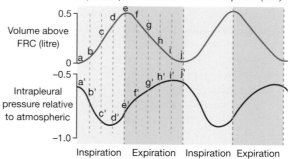

Inspiration   Expiration   Inspiration   Expiration

Figure 6c Surface tension

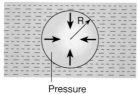

Pressure above ambient = P

Laplace's equation

$$P= \frac{2T}{R}$$

T= Surface tension

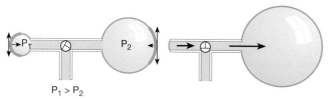

$P_1 > P_2$

∴ When tap is opened the small bubble empties into the large

Figure 6d Effect of surface area

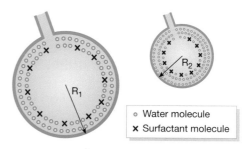

○ Water molecule
✕ Surfactant molecule

$R_2 < R_1$ but $T_2 < T_1$ because surface concentration of surfactant is higher when the alveolus is small
The fall in R is more than offset by the fall in T,
∴ since $P = \frac{2T}{R}$, P does not rise, but falls as the alveolus shrinks

The Respiratory System at a Glance, Fourth Edition. Jeremy P.T. Ward. © Jeremy P.T. Ward. Published 2015 by John Wiley & Sons, Ltd.

To breathe in, the inspiratory muscles must contract to overcome the impedance offered by the lungs and chest wall. This is mainly in the form of frictional **airway resistance** (Chapter 7) and **elastic resistance** to stretching of the lung and chest wall tissues and the fluid lining the alveoli. Chest wall diseases, such as kyphoscoliosis or scarring following burns, can increase respiratory system elastic resistance but these conditions are usually obvious; lung stiffness is more common and its assessment requires lung function tests.

Assessing the stiffness of the lungs: lung compliance

The 'stretchiness' of the lung is usually assessed as lung compliance (C_L), which is the change in lung volume per unit change in distending pressure ($C_L = \Delta v / \Delta P$). The distending pressure, P, is the pressure difference across the lung, which equals alveolar–intrapleural pressure. Lung compliance is the inverse of elastic resistance; stiff lungs have high elastic resistance or low compliance.

Intrapleural pressure can be assessed by measuring oesophageal pressure (Chapter 3). Alveolar pressure cannot easily be measured directly, but when no air is flowing, alveolar pressure must equal mouth pressure (i.e. zero). The transmural pressure, P, is then equal to intrapleural pressure. The subject breathes in steps and measurements are taken while the breath is held and plotted as a **static pressure–volume (P–V) curve** (Fig. 6a). The curve flattens as the lung volume approaches total lung capacity (TLC). The inspiratory curve is slightly different from the expiratory curve, and this **hysteresis** is a common property of elastic bodies. **Static lung compliance** is the slope of the steepest part of this static P–V curve in the region just above functional residual capacity (FRC).

Lung compliance is normally about 1.5 L/kPa, but as with lung volumes it is affected by the subject's size, age and gender. In **restrictive disease**, such as lung fibrosis, lung compliance is low. Like a stiff spring, once stretched, fibrosed lungs have an increased tendency to shrink back to their resting position or increased **elastic recoil**. The loss of alveolar tissue in **emphysema** makes them easier to stretch and lung compliance is increased. Although safe, swallowing an oesophageal balloon is not very pleasant or convenient. Fortunately, it is often possible to deduce that a patient has stiff lungs from other measurements such as **TLC**, **FRC** (Chapters 3, 22 and 32), forced expiratory volume in 1 second (**FEV$_1$**) and forced vital capacity (**FVC**) (Chapter 22).

Dynamic pressure–volume loops and dynamic compliance

A **dynamic P–V loop** (upper panel of Fig. 6b) is obtained from continuous measurements of intrapleural pressure and volume during a normal breathing cycle (lower panel of Fig. 6b). There are two points, at the ends of inspiration and expiration, where airflow and alveolar pressure are zero (a, a' and e', e') and the slope of the line joining these points is **dynamic compliance**. In health, its value is similar to the **static compliance**, but in some diseases it may be lower, as stiff areas may fill preferentially during normal breathing. Between the two zero flow points, the dynamic P–V loop appears fatter than the static P–V loop, as intrapleural pressure must change more to drive airflow. In fact, the area of the dynamic loop is a measure of the work done against airway resistance (Chapter 7).

The air–fluid interface lining the alveoli

During inspiration, as well as stretching the collagen and elastin fibres, the **surface tension** forces at the air–alveolar lining fluid interface must be overcome. At the surface of a bubble, the attraction of the fluid molecules for each other creates a tension, which tends to shrink the bubble (Fig. 6c). Laplace discovered that a gas bubble in a liquid would shrink until the pressure, P, within which it reached a value of $2T/R$, where T is a constant, the surface tension of the fluid, and R is the radius of the bubble. When a bubble has air on both sides, there are two air–fluid interfaces and $P = 4T/R$. The **law of Laplace** ($P = 2T/R$ or $4T/R$) predicts that, if two bubbles are made of the same fluid, the smaller bubble will have a higher pressure within it – since when the radius of curvature is small, a greater proportion of the surface tension is directed to the centre of the bubble (lower panel of Fig. 6c). When the two bubbles are connected, the small bubble empties into the large bubble as air flows down the pressure gradient.

The lungs are not a simple system of bubbles connected by tubes but much more complicated. In life alveoli are not spherical, they have interconnections between neighbouring alveoli and alveolar fluid may not produce a continuous lining to the alveoli. Nevertheless, the surface tension forces illustrated by this model are undoubtedly important in the lung and the presence of an air–fluid interface creates several potential problems:

1 It reduces lung compliance and the higher the surface tension the lower the compliance.
2 The alveoli and small airways would be inherently unstable, tending to collapse under surface tension forces during expiration resulting in areas of **atelectasis**.

The absence of these problems in healthy humans is thought to be partly due to the presence in the alveolar lining fluid of **surfactant**.

Surfactant

Pulmonary surfactant is a mixture of **phospholipids**, such as phosphatidylcholine and proteins, produced by the **type II pneumocytes** (Chapter 5). The presence of these substances in the **alveolar lining fluid** lowers the surface tension and increases compliance. The phospholipids have a **hydrophilic** end that lies in the alveolar fluid and a **hydrophobic** end that projects into the alveolar gas, and as a result they float on the surface of the lining fluid. As an alveolus shrinks, its surface area diminishes and the surface concentration of surfactant rises (Fig. 6d). As surface tension falls with increasing surface concentration of surfactant, the increased tendency for alveoli to collapse when they shrink is offset and stability is improved. Alveolar stability is also aided by the connection and mutual pull of neighbouring alveoli, a phenomenon known as **alveolar interdependence**.

Surfactant production in the fetus gradually increases in the last third of pregnancy and may be inadequate in babies born prematurely, giving rise to the typical problems of **neonatal respiratory distress syndrome (NRDS)** – stiff lungs and areas of collapse leading to increased work of breathing and reduced gas exchange (Chapters 17 and 18).

Surfactant proteins (e.g. SP-A, SP-B, SP-C and SP-D) contribute to the surface tension lowering actions of phospholipids, as well as having other functions such as host defence. They are probably the reason why natural (animal-derived) surfactant preparations have proved more effective for treating NRDS than artificial surfactant composed only of phospholipids. Artificial surfactant protein analogues are being introduced in the hope of improving the non-animal preparations.

7 Lung mechanics: airway resistance

Figure 7a Laminar and turbulent flow

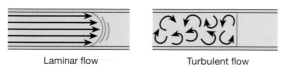

Laminar flow   Turbulent flow

Figure 7b Main factors influencing bronchomotor tone

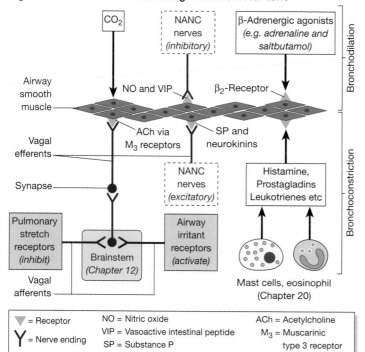

CO_2 NANC nerves *(inhibitory)*   β-Adrenergic agonists *(e.g. adrenaline and saltbutamol)*

Bronchodilation

Airway smooth muscle

NO and VIP β_2-Receptor

ACh via M_3 receptors   SP and neurokinins

Vagal efferents

Synapse

NANC nerves *(excitatory)*

Histamine, Prostagladins Leukotrienes etc

Bronchoconstriction

Pulmonary stretch receptors *(inhibit)*

Airway irritant receptors *(activate)*

Brainstem *(Chapter 12)*

Vagal afferents

Mast cells, eosinophil (Chapter 20)

▼ = Receptor   NO = Nitric oxide   ACh = Acetylcholine
Y = Nerve ending   VIP = Vasoactive intestinal peptide M_3 = Muscarinic
   SP = Substance P   type 3 receptor

Figure 7d Dynamic compression of airways

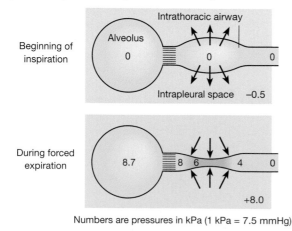

Beginning of inspiration

Intrathoracic airway

Alveolus

0

0   0

Intrapleural space   −0.5

During forced expiration

8.7

8   6   4   0

+8.0

Numbers are pressures in kPa (1 kPa = 7.5 mmHg)

Figure 7c The effect of effort on inspiratory and expiratory airflow

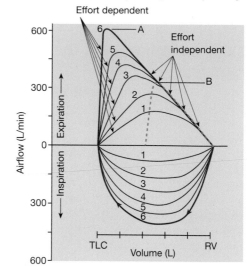

Effort dependent

Effort independent

A

B

Airflow (L/min)

Expiration

Inspiration

TLC   Volume (L)   RV

- - - - = Flow–volume curve for maximum effort from partly filled lungs
A = Peak expiratory flow rate with lungs filled to total lung capacity,
B = Peak expiratory flow rate for partly filled lungs filled (RV + 3 L),
TLC = Total lung capacity, RV = Residual volume

Figure 7e Maximum flow–volume loops

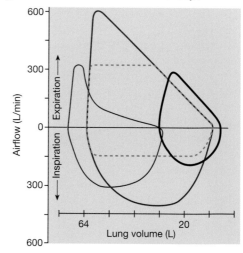

Airflow (L/min)

Expiration

Inspiration

64   20

Lung volume (L)

—— **Normal curve**

—— **Obstructive airway disease of smaller airways.** Note:
 • Concave appearance of forced expiratory curve
 • Forced inspiratory flow affected less than forced expiratory flow

- - - **Upper airway obstruction (e.g. tracheal stenosis).** Note:
 • Flat topped flow–volume curve
 • Forced inspiratory flow affected as much as expiratory flow

—— **Restrictive lung disease.** Low peak flow rates are related to low volume. (Note: this figure is drawn to show the relationship between these traces by using absolute lung volume which cannot actually be obtained from a flow–volume loop alone).

The Respiratory System at a Glance, Fourth Edition. Jeremy P.T. Ward. © Jeremy P.T. Ward. Published 2015 by John Wiley & Sons, Ltd.

Airflow is driven by the mouth–alveolar pressure gradient generated by the respiratory muscles (Chapters 2 and 3).

$$Airflow \frac{\Delta P(= mouth - alveolar\ pressure)}{RAW(= resistance\ of\ the\ airways)}$$

In **laminar flow**, gas particles move parallel to the walls, with centre layers moving faster than outer ones, creating a cone-shaped front (Fig. 7a). The factors affecting laminar flow of a fluid of viscosity, η, in smooth straight tubes of length, l, and radius, r, are described in **Poiseuille's equation**:

$$Flow = \frac{\Delta P}{R} = \Delta P \frac{\pi r^4}{8\ell\eta} \quad \therefore R = \frac{8\ell\eta}{\pi r^4}$$

Halving the radius of an airway increases its resistance 16-fold. However, although the resistance of an individual bronchiole is high, there are thousands in parallel. The total resistance of each generation of peripheral airways is normally low, and the overall resistance of lung airways is dominated by the larger airways. Outside the lung, the nose and pharynx contribute substantial resistance, which can be reduced by mouth breathing, for example, during exercise. Peripheral airways are often affected by disease, but because their resistance must increase considerably to measurably affect airway resistance (RAW), they are known as the **silent zone**.

At higher linear velocities, especially in wide airways and near branch points, flow may become **turbulent**. With turbulence, the wave front is square and flow $\propto \sqrt{\Delta P}$ (not ΔP), reflecting the dissipation of energy in the formation of eddies. Normally, at rest, flow is laminar throughout the airways, but in exercise it may become turbulent, especially in the trachea, generating characteristic harsh breath sounds.

Factors affecting airway resistance

Bronchial smooth muscle and epithelium

Bronchial smooth muscle (Fig. 7b) receives a **parasympathetic bronchoconstrictor** nerve supply, acting via acetylcholine and muscarinic type 3 receptors, which forms the efferent limb of a reflex from airway irritant receptors (rapidly adapting receptors). The smooth muscle also contains β_2-adrenergic receptors, which cause relaxation when stimulated by circulating **epinephrine** (adrenaline) or drugs such as salbutamol. Sympathetic innervation of the airways is sparse in humans and has little effect on airway smooth muscle. Airways are also supplied with excitatory and inhibitory non-adrenergic non-cholinergic (NANC) nerves, the former acting via the transmitters substance P and neurokinins, and the latter via nitric oxide (NO) and/or vasoactive intestinal peptide (VIP). Parasympathetic bronchoconstriction is inhibited by activation of airway slowly adapting stretch receptors. CO_2 has a direct bronchodilator effect. Pollutants (e.g. sulphur dioxide and ozone) and substances released from mast cells and eosinophils can increase RAW via bronchoconstriction, mucosal oedema, mucus hypersecretion, mucus plugging and epithelial shedding – all of which are important in asthma (Chapter 26). Increased airway resistance can also be caused by chronic mucosal hypertrophy in chronic obstructive pulmonary disease (COPD) (Chapter 28) and by material within the airways, such as inhaled foreign bodies or tumours (Chapter 42).

Transmural (airway-intrapleural) pressure gradient

The pressure difference across airways can have important effects on their calibre, and this underlies the effects of effort on airflow, illustrated in Figure 7c. Airflow is measured continuously and plotted against lung volume as the subject breathes between residual volume (RV) and total lung capacity (TLC). The inspiratory airflow at any volume increases progressively with increasing effort (1 = minimum effort, 6 = maximum effort). The flow–volume curves for progressively increasing expiratory efforts (upper traces 1–6) are more complicated. In the early part of expiration from TLC, flow is **effort dependent**, but towards the end of the breath, as volume declines, the traces produced at different effort levels come together. Expiratory airflow towards the end of a breath is **effort independent** and determined by lung volume. **Peak expiratory flow rate** (PEFR) is seen to be reduced (B in Fig. 7c) if the lungs are only partially filled at the start of the forced expiration. Effort-independent airflow is explained by **dynamic compression of airways**. Before the start of inspiration (Fig. 7d, upper panel) the pressure along the airways is zero, intrapleural pressure is negative (Chapter 3) and transmural pressure acts to hold airways open. Intrapleural pressure is negative during both quiet and forced inspiration and it remains negative in quiet expiration, so transmural pressure holds airways open. In a forced expiration, however, expiratory muscle contraction raises intrapleural pressure well above atmospheric pressure (e.g. 8 kPa, 60 mmHg), increasing the pressure gradient from alveoli to mouth. This would be expected to increase airflow, but the increased intrapleural pressure also acts to compress airways. Airway pressure falls progressively along the airway, and at some point – usually in the bronchi – the airway pressure will be sufficiently below intrapleural pressure for the airway to collapse, despite its cartilaginous support. Pressure will then build up distally, opening the airways again. The resulting fluttering walls can be seen during bronchoscopy; they produce the brassy note audible on forced expiration in healthy people.

RAW in disease

Increased airway resistance is important in many diseases and can be measured using a body plethysmograph. In healthy individuals, RAW is about 0.2 kPa/L per second (1.5 mmHg/L per second). More commonly, airway resistance is assessed indirectly from forced expiratory measurements, such as **forced expiratory volume in 1 second** (FEV$_1$), **forced vital capacity** (FVC) and PEFR (Chapter 22). Especially useful is the **forced expiratory ratio** (FER = FEV$_1$/FVC), which is reduced when RAW is increased in **obstructive pulmonary disease**. High airway resistance accentuates dynamic compression of airways by augmenting the pressure drop along airways. In addition, the airways may be less able to resist compression in emphysema because of reduced radial traction and in asthma because of bronchoconstriction. Collapse of small airways may occur, leading to incomplete expiration (**air trapping**) and increased functional residual capacity. Inability to produce high expiratory airflow impairs effective coughing, which can lead to a vicious cycle as secretions accumulate, further increasing RAW and further reducing peak flow. **Expiratory wheezes (rhonchi)**, heard in asthma and other obstructive diseases, are probably generated by oscillations in opposing airway walls near their point of closure, like sounds from the reeds of an oboe. A reasonable airflow is needed to generate such sounds, and when constriction becomes very severe, they disappear to give the ominous silent chest seen in life-threatening asthma. Small airway collapse leads to characteristic shape of the maximum flow–volume curve in obstructive airway disease (Fig. 7e), which differs from that in upper airway obstruction and restrictive lung disease.

8 Carriage of oxygen

Figure 8a Haemoglobin structure

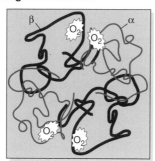

Haemoglobin is composed of four subunits, each containing a protein chain (globin) and a haem group. Normal adult haemoglobin, HbA, contains two identical α-chains composed of 141 amino acids and two β-chains composed of 146 amino acids. The haem group ( ) is attached to each chain at a histidine residue, and each has an iron atom in the ferrous form, which binds to an oxygen molecule. The haem groups lie in crevices in the crumpled ball of globin chains. The exact 3D (or quaternary) structure of haemoglobin can change and alter the accessibility of the oxygen-binding site. Each molecule of haemoglobin can bind up to four molecules of oxygen in a series of reactions which can be summarized as:

$$Hb_4 + 4O_2 \Leftrightarrow Hb_4(O_2)_4$$

Figure 8b The oxygen–haemoglobin dissociation curve, haemoglobin concentration (150 g/L)

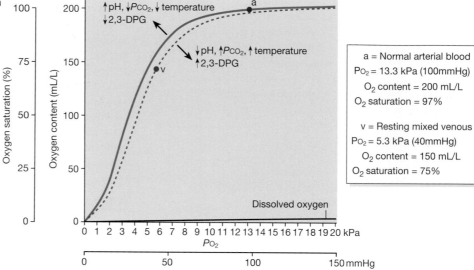

a = Normal arterial blood
P_{O_2} = 13.3 kPa (100 mmHg)
O_2 content = 200 mL/L
O_2 saturation = 97%

v = Resting mixed venous
P_{O_2} = 5.3 kPa (40 mmHg)
O_2 content = 150 mL/L
O_2 saturation = 75%

Figure 8c Anaemia and carbon monoxide poisoning

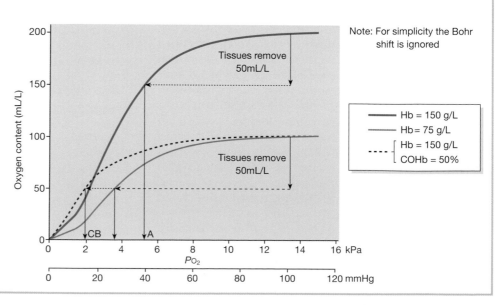

Note: For simplicity the Bohr shift is ignored

—— Hb = 150 g/L
—— Hb = 75 g/L
- - - Hb = 150 g/L
      COHb = 50%

The Respiratory System at a Glance, Fourth Edition. Jeremy P.T. Ward. © Jeremy P.T. Ward. Published 2015 by John Wiley & Sons, Ltd.

At rest, a man consumes about 250 mL oxygen per minute, which may rise to more than 4000 mL/min in exercise if he is very fit. Oxygen diffuses from alveolus to blood until equilibrium is reached when pulmonary capillary P_{O_2} equals alveolar P_{O_2}. The **solubility** of oxygen in blood is low – 0.000225 mL oxygen per mL of blood per kPa (0.00003 mL/mL per mmHg) – so that at a normal arterial P_{O_2} of 13.3 kPa (100 mmHg) there is only 3 mL dissolved in each litre of blood. The main function of the red blood cell pigment, **haemoglobin**, the key features of whose structure is shown in Figure 8a, is to carry the large quantities of oxygen needed by the tissues.

Each gram of haemoglobin combines with up to 1.34 mL oxygen, so with a haemoglobin concentration, [Hb], of 150 g/L, blood contains a maximum of 200 mL/L oxygen bound to haemoglobin. This is known as the **oxygen capacity**, which varies with [Hb]. The percentage of binding sites which are actually bound to oxygen, the **oxygen saturation,** depends on the P_{O_2} to which the haemoglobin is exposed.

Oxygen saturation:

$$\frac{\text{Amount of oxygen bound to haemoglobin (mL/L)}}{\text{Oxygen capacity (mL/L)}} \times 100\%$$

The oxygen content of the blood (mL/L) equals the sum of haemoglobin-bound oxygen and the small amount of dissolved oxygen. The rate of rise of oxygen content with increasing partial pressure depends on the number of free haemoglobin-binding sites remaining and their affinity for oxygen. Haemoglobin exists in two different quaternary states, 'tense' when it is deoxygenated and 'relaxed' when it is oxygenated. As each oxygen molecule binds in turn to the four haem groups, the quaternary structure alters and the affinity of the remaining binding sites for oxygen increases. This **cooperative binding** increases the steepness of the **oxygen-haemoglobin dissociation curve** in the middle (Fig. 8b); the curve flattens again when P_{O_2} is above about 8 kPa (60 mmHg) because there are few unfilled binding sites remaining. In arterial blood, P_{O_2} is normally about 13 kPa (100 mmHg), oxygen saturation about 97%, and with a normal [Hb], oxygen content is about 200 mL/L. Rises or modest falls in P_{O_2} from 13 kPa (100 mmHg), for example, during hyperventilation or mild hypoventilation, cause little change in the arterial oxygen content, as the dissociation curve is flat in this region. More severe reductions in P_{O_2}, to levels in the steep region (<8 kPa, 60 mmHg), are associated with significant reductions in oxygen saturation and content. Consequently, breathing oxygen-enriched air may significantly raise arterial oxygen content and exercise capacity at high altitude and in patients with chronic hypoxic respiratory disease, but it has little effect in a healthy person at sea level.

Low P_{O_2} in tissue capillaries causes oxygen release from haemoglobin, whereas the high P_{O_2} in pulmonary capillaries causes oxygen binding. The affinity of haemoglobin for oxygen varies with local conditions. A reduced oxygen affinity, shown by a right shift in the curve, is caused by a fall in pH, a rise in P_{CO_2} (the **Bohr effect**) or increased temperature (Fig. 8b). These changes occur in metabolically active tissues such as exercising muscle and encourage oxygen release. In the lungs, oxygen uptake is aided by the increased affinity of haemoglobin for oxygen (left-shifted dissociation curve), caused by the lower P_{CO_2} and temperature and increased pH. The P_{O_2} at which the haemoglobin is 50% saturated is known as the P_{50}. Under normal arterial conditions (pH = 7.4, P_{CO_2} = 5.3 kPa or 40 mmHg, temperature = 37°C) P_{50}= 3.5 kPa (26.3 mmHg); right shifts raise the P_{50} and left shifts lower it. A rise in the concentration of **2,3-di(or bi)phosphoglycerate** (2,3-DPG), which is a by-product of glycolysis in red cells, also causes a right shift. A rise in 2,3-DPG occurs in anaemia, causing a modest increase in P_{50}. Blood bank storage causes progressive depletion of 2,3-DPG and an undesirable left shift, but this can be minimized by storing the blood with citrate-phosphate-dextrose.

Anaemia and carbon monoxide poisoning

In **anaemia**, at any given P_{O_2}, the oxygen content is reduced because of the reduced concentration of binding sites. Figure 8c shows the dissociation curve for normal blood and for blood with [Hb] = 75 g/L. Alveolar and arterial P_{O_2} is normal in anaemia and therefore arterial O_2 content is 100 mL/L. At rest, the tissues need to remove about 50 mL/L of oxygen from the blood passing through them. To achieve this mixed venous P_{O_2} will need to fall to about 5.3 kPa (40 mmHg) (A in Fig. 8c) when [Hb] = 150 g/L and about 3.6 kPa (27 mmHg) (B) when [Hb] = 75 g/L. The reduced venous and hence capillary P_{O_2} reduces the partial pressure gradient driving diffusion of oxygen to the tissues, which is adequate at rest but which may become inadequate in exercise when oxygen consumption increases.

Figure 8c also shows the dissociation curve for blood that has 50% of oxygen-binding sites occupied by carbon monoxide (CO, dashed line). Arterial oxygen content is 100 mL/L, but there is also an altered shape and leftward shift of the dissociation curve, because CO binding increases the affinity of the remaining (CO-free) sites for oxygen. This impairs oxygen release in the tissues. Mixed venous P_{O_2} will now have to fall to 2 kPa (15 mmHg) (point C) to release the 50 mL/L required, and this will greatly reduce the pressure gradient for diffusion. At about 50–60% **carboxyhaemoglobin**, symptoms of impaired cerebral oxygenation (headache, convulsions, coma and death) are severe, whereas anaemic patients with the same arterial oxygen content are typically asymptomatic at rest. Haemoglobin has a high affinity for CO (~240 times that for oxygen), so breathing even at low concentrations causes a progressive increase in the cherry-red carboxyhaemoglobin. A cherry-red complexion is sometimes a feature of CO poisoning, although pallor and **cyanosis** (discussed in Chapter 25) are more common.

Other respiratory pigments

Fetal haemoglobin, HbF, differs from **adult haemoglobin, HbA,** in that there are two γ-chains instead of two β-chains. The HbF dissociation curve lies to the left of that for HbA, reflecting its higher O_2 affinity. This difference is enhanced by the **double Bohr shift**: in the placenta P_{CO_2} moves from the fetal to maternal blood, shifting the maternal curve further right and the fetal curve further left. The high affinity of HbF relative to HbA helps transfer oxygen from mother to fetus, and even though blood returning from the placenta to the fetus in the umbilical vein has a P_{O_2} of only about 4 kPa (30 mmHg), its saturation is 70%. Oxygen transport in the fetus is also helped by a high [Hb] of about 170–180 g/L.

Myoglobin, the respiratory pigment found in muscle, is composed of a single haem group attached to a single globin chain. With no cooperative binding, its dissociation curve is hyperbolic. It is also far to the left of HbA and its high affinity means that its oxygen store is only released when local P_{O_2} is severely reduced, for example in heavy exercise.

9 Carriage of carbon dioxide

Figure 9a Carriage of CO₂ at rest

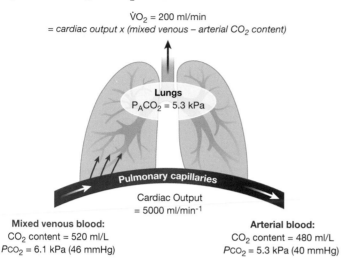

$\dot{V}O_2 = 200$ ml/min
= cardiac output x (mixed venous – arterial CO₂ content)

Lungs
$P_ACO_2 = 5.3$ kPa

Pulmonary capillaries

Cardiac Output
= 5000 ml/min⁻¹

Mixed venous blood:
CO_2 content = 520 ml/L
$PCO_2 = 6.1$ kPa (46 mmHg)

Arterial blood:
CO_2 content = 480 ml/L
$PCO_2 = 5.3$ kPa (40 mmHg)

Figure 9c How CO₂ is carried in arterial and venous blood

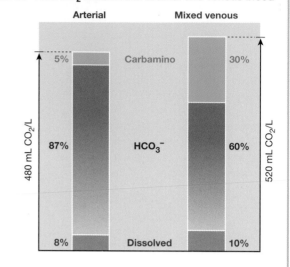

Figure 9b CO₂ dissociation curve

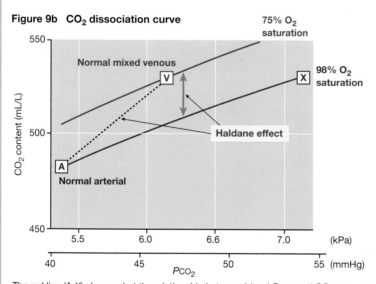

The basis of the Haldane effect

When haemoglobin is fully oxygenated, each of the four Hb subunits is bound to one O_2: $Hb_4(O_2)_4$
As O_2 is released, i.e.

$$Hb_4(O_2)_4 \longrightarrow Hb_4(O_2)_3 \longrightarrow Hb_4(O_2)_2 \longrightarrow Hb_4(O_2)$$

the ability of each reduced (deoxygenated) Hb subunit (H•Hb) to buffer H^+ and form Hb•COOH (carbaminohaemoglobin) is greatly increased

This enhances carriage of CO_2 by blood by:
  (a) buffering red cell acidity and therefore facilitating formation of HCO_3^-
  (b) formation of Hb•COOH

When blood is reoxygenated in the lungs, the reverse occurs, facilitating removal of CO_2 in the breath

The red line (A-X) shows what the relationship between blood PCO_2 and CO_2 content would be if Hb remained 98% saturated. However, as mixed venous blood HB is only 75% saturated, more CO_2 can be carried for any given PCO_2, as shown by the dashed line A-V (the Haldane effect, see box and text).

Figure 9d CO₂ uptake and O₂ delivery in the tissues – role of red cells

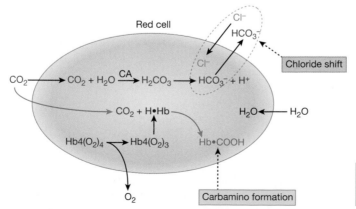

CA = carbonic anhydrase
Hb = haemoglobin subunit
H•Hb = reduced haemoglobin

Carbon dioxide (CO_2) is produced by tissues and transported in the blood to the lungs, where it is expired. About 40% of the venous CO_2 delivered to the lungs is expired in the breath at rest (Fig. 9a). The amount of CO_2 that can be carried in the blood is much greater than that of O_2, as seen in the **CO_2 dissociation curve** (Fig. 9b). This is also more linear than that for O_2 and does not reach a plateau. CO_2 is transported in the blood as bicarbonate ions, as carbamino compounds combined with proteins or simply dissolved in the plasma (Fig. 9c).

Bicarbonate: In mixed venous blood about 60% of CO_2 is transported in the form of bicarbonate. CO_2 and water combine to form carbonic acid (H_2CO_3) and thence bicarbonate (HCO_3^-):

$$CO_2 + H_2O \overset{CA}{\Leftrightarrow} H_2CO_3 \Leftrightarrow H^+ + HCO_3^- \tag{1}$$

The left-hand side of the equation proceeds slowly in plasma, but is accelerated dramatically by the enzyme **carbonic anhydrase** (CA), which is present in red blood cells. Ionization of carbonic acid to bicarbonate and H^+ is rapid in the absence of any enzyme. Bicarbonate is therefore formed preferentially in the red cells, from which it easily diffuses out into the plasma. The red cell membrane is however impermeable to H^+ ions and they remain within the cell. To maintain electrical neutrality, Cl^- ions diffuse into the cell to replace bicarbonate, an effect known as the **chloride shift** (Fig. 9c). A build-up of H^+ in the red blood cell would impair further movement of Equation 1 to the right, thus limiting formation of bicarbonate. However, H^+ binds avidly to reduced (deoxygenated) haemoglobin; that is, **haemoglobin acts as a buffer**, so the rise in H^+ concentration is limited and more bicarbonate can be formed. Oxygenated haemoglobin does not bind H^+ as well, as it is more acidic. This contributes to the **Haldane effect**, which states that, for any given P_{CO_2}, the CO_2 content of deoxygenated blood is greater than that of oxygenated blood. As a result, when blood gives up oxygen to respiring tissues, that is, becomes deoxygenated, it is able to take up more of the CO_2 that the tissues are producing. Conversely, oxygenation of haemoglobin in the lung assists the unloading of CO_2 from the blood so that it can be expired. This is illustrated in Figure 9b and Equation 2.

$$H^+ + haemoglobin \cdot O_2 \Leftrightarrow haemoglobin \cdot H + O_2 \tag{2}$$

Note that as a consequence of all the above, deoxygenated red blood cells have a higher intracellular osmolality and water enters, causing them to swell slightly. In the lung, CO_2 is given off, osmolality falls and the red cells shrink again.

Carbamino compounds: CO_2 combines rapidly with terminal amino groups on proteins to form carbamino compounds:

$$CO_2 + protein \cdot NH_2 \Leftrightarrow protein \cdot NH \cdot COOH \tag{3}$$

The most prevalent protein in blood is haemoglobin, which combines with CO_2 to form carbaminohaemoglobin. Reduced haemoglobin forms carbamino compounds more readily than oxygenated haemoglobin, and this also contributes to the Haldane effect (Fig. 9b). About 30% of the CO_2 expired is carried to the lungs as carbamino compounds.

CO_2 in solution: CO_2 is approximately 20 times more soluble in water than O_2. A significant proportion (~10%) of the CO_2 exhaled is therefore carried to the lung dissolved in the plasma.

Because of the Haldane effect, the proportion of CO_2 that is carried in the blood as bicarbonate, carbamino compounds and simply dissolved differs between oxygenated arterial blood and deoxygenated mixed venous blood (Fig. 9c).

Hypoventilation and hyperventilation

Ventilation is normally closely matched to the metabolic requirements of the body, and this can be estimated from the rate of CO_2 production (Chapter 12). The partial pressure of CO_2 in the alveoli ($P_{A}CO_2$) is proportional to the amount of CO_2 exhaled per minute (V_{CO_2}) as a fraction of total alveolar ventilation (V_A), that is, $P_{A}CO_2 \propto V_{CO_2}/V_A$. The gas in the alveoli is in equilibrium with arterial blood, so $P_{A}CO_2$ estimates the partial pressure in the blood ($P_{a}CO_2$). At any given metabolic rate, doubling the alveolar ventilation halves alveolar and arterial P_{CO_2}, and halving alveolar ventilation doubles $P_{A}CO_2$ and $P_{a}CO_2$. Changes in alveolar ventilation also affect alveolar P_{O_2}, but the relationship is not as simple because O_2 is present in both inspired and expired gas. Thus, doubling alveolar ventilation will halve the *difference* between the inspired and alveolar O_2 fraction. **Hypoventilation** (underventilation) and **hyperventilation** (overventilation) are therefore defined in terms of $P_{a}CO_2$, so that a patient is *hypoventilating* when $P_{a}CO_2$ is more than 45 mmHg (5.9 kPa) and *hyperventilating* when the $P_{a}CO_2$ is less than 40 mmHg (5.3 kPa). Note that the CO_2 content of the blood will be affected more slowly by hypo- or hyperventilation than the O_2 content, as the CO_2 stores in the body (e.g. as HCO_3^-) are approximately 75 times greater than those for O_2 (e.g. haemoglobin and myoglobin). Also, although hyperventilation increases arterial P_{O_2}, in a healthy patient it has little effect on O_2 content as arterial haemoglobin is normally close to saturation (Chapter 8).

Hypoventilation may occur when the respiratory drive is impaired by head injury, or drugs such as morphine or barbiturates which suppress the respiratory centres. It may also be caused by respiratory muscle weakness or severe chest trauma. Hypoventilation is sometimes a feature of severe chronic obstructive airways disease (COPD; Chapter 28) or obesity (obesity hypoventilation syndrome; Chapter 46), but is not usually a feature of asthma (Chapter 27) unless the attack is severe or prolonged enough to lead to exhaustion. Hypoventilation is difficult to achieve voluntarily, as the respiratory centres create an overwhelming desire to breathe.

Hypoventilation leads to **hypercapnia** (high $P_{a}CO_2$) and **hypoxia** (low $P_{a}O_2$). Increasing severity of hypercapnia causes peripheral vasodilatation, muscle twitching and hand flap, confusion, drowsiness and eventually coma; there is a concomitant respiratory acidosis (Chapter 10). The effects of hypoxia are dealt with elsewhere (Chapter 8). Hyperventilation can be induced voluntarily and in states of high anxiety (e.g. panic attacks) or pain. It results in a low $P_{a}CO_2$ (**hypocapnia**), which can cause light-headedness, visual disturbances due to cerebral vasoconstriction, paraesthesia ('pins and needles') and muscle cramps, especially carpopedal spasm; there is a concomitant respiratory alkalosis (Chapter 10).

Respiratory gas exchange ratio

Respiratory gas exchange ratio (R) is the ratio of CO_2 production to O_2 consumption as measured at the mouth. In the steady state, CO_2 production and O_2 consumption reflect tissue metabolism. Metabolizing carbohydrates produces a volume of CO_2 equal to the volume of O_2 consumed, whereas metabolizing fats and proteins produces a smaller volume of CO_2 than O_2 consumed. For an average mixed diet $R \approx 0.8$.

10 Acid–base balance

Figure 10a pH range and examples

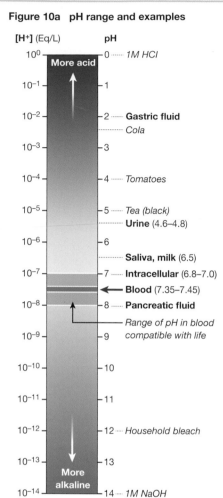

[H+] (Eq/L)   pH

$[H^+]$ (Eq/L)	pH	
10^0	0	1M HCl
More acid		
10^{-1}	1	
10^{-2}	2	**Gastric fluid**
		Cola
10^{-3}	3	
10^{-4}	4	Tomatoes
10^{-5}	5	Tea (black)
		Urine (4.6–4.8)
10^{-6}	6	
		Saliva, milk (6.5)
10^{-7}	7	**Intracellular (6.8–7.0)**
		Blood (7.35–7.45)
10^{-8}	8	**Pancreatic fluid**
		Range of pH in blood compatible with life
10^{-9}	9	
10^{-10}	10	
10^{-11}	11	
10^{-12}	12	Household bleach
10^{-13}	13	
More alkaline		
10^{-14}	14	1M NaOH

Figure 10e Key physiological buffers

Blood	Bicarbonate Haemoglobin Plasma proteins (minor) (too little phosphate to be effective)
Interstitial fluid	Bicarbonate (very little protein) (too little phosphate to be effective)
Intracellular fluid	Proteins Phosphate (little bicarbonate)
Urine	Phosphate Ammonia (prevents excessive acidity, 'traps' H+ in tubular fluid)
Saliva	Bicarbonate, but HCO₃⁻ actively secreted by gland to prevent excessive acidity

Figure 10b Acid-base balance

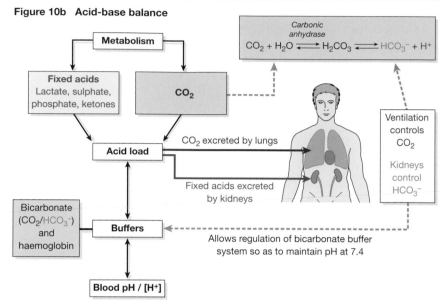

Metabolism

Fixed acids
Lactate, sulphate, phosphate, ketones

CO₂

Carbonic anhydrase
$CO_2 + H_2O \rightleftharpoons H_2CO_3 \rightleftharpoons HCO_3^- + H^+$

Acid load

CO₂ excreted by lungs

Fixed acids excreted by kidneys

Ventilation controls CO₂

Kidneys control HCO₃⁻

Bicarbonate (CO₂/HCO₃⁻) and haemoglobin

Buffers

Allows regulation of bicarbonate buffer system so as to maintain pH at 7.4

Blood pH / [H+]

Figure 10c Buffers, weak acids and the Henderson-Hasselbalch equation

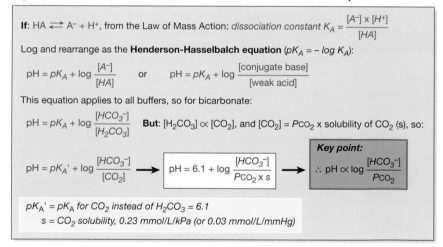

If: $HA \rightleftharpoons A^- + H^+$, from the Law of Mass Action: dissociation constant $K_A = \dfrac{[A^-] \times [H^+]}{[HA]}$

Log and rearrange as the **Henderson-Hasselbalch equation** ($pK_A = -log\ K_A$):

$$pH = pK_A + \log \frac{[A^-]}{[HA]} \quad \text{or} \quad pH = pK_A + \log \frac{[\text{conjugate base}]}{[\text{weak acid}]}$$

This equation applies to all buffers, so for bicarbonate:

$$pH = pK_A + \log \frac{[HCO_3^-]}{[H_2CO_3]} \quad \textbf{But}: [H_2CO_3] \propto [CO_2], \text{ and } [CO_2] = PCO_2 \times \text{solubility of } CO_2 \text{ (s), so:}$$

$$pH = pK_A' + \log \frac{[HCO_3^-]}{[CO_2]} \longrightarrow pH = 6.1 + \log \frac{[HCO_3^-]}{PCO_2 \times s} \longrightarrow$$

Key point:
$$\therefore pH \propto \log \frac{[HCO_3^-]}{PCO_2}$$

$pK_A' = pK_A$ for CO_2 instead of $H_2CO_3 = 6.1$
$s = CO_2$ solubility, 0.23 mmol/L/kPa (or 0.03 mmol/L/mmHg)

Figure 10d Buffer (titration) curve: Effect of addition of acid or alkali on pH of a bicarbonate buffered solution

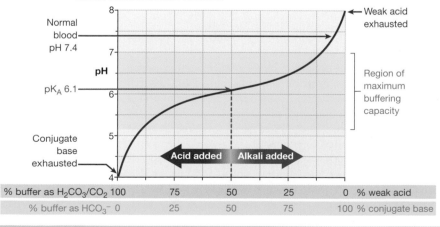

Weak acid exhausted

Normal blood pH 7.4

pKₐ 6.1

Region of maximum buffering capacity

pH

Conjugate base exhausted

Acid added   Alkali added

| % buffer as H₂CO₃/CO₂ | 100 | 75 | 50 | 25 | 0 | % weak acid |
| % buffer as HCO₃⁻ | 0 | 25 | 50 | 75 | 100 | % conjugate base |

The Respiratory System at a Glance, Fourth Edition. Jeremy P.T. Ward. © Jeremy P.T. Ward. Published 2015 by John Wiley & Sons, Ltd.

The concentration of H$^+$ in a solution (i.e. acidity or alkalinity) is commonly expressed in terms of pH, the negative log of [H$^+$]. Whilst intracellular pH is most important for tissue function, clinical assessment of **acid–base status** is most easily obtained from blood analysis. The pH of arterial blood is normally maintained within a narrow range, **7.35–7.45** (45–35 nmol/L) (Fig. 10a). A pH less than 7.35 is termed **acidosis**, and greater than 7.45 **alkalosis**, both of which can have serious consequences. A pH outside the range of 7.0–7.8 may be fatal.

Sources of acid

Some acid is ingested with food, but most arises from metabolism, and production and transport of CO_2. CO_2 is not an acid, but acts like one because it spontaneously combines with water to form **carbonic acid** (H_2CO_3), a process facilitated by **carbonic anhydrase**; CO_2 and H_2CO_3 are thus in equilibrium. H_2CO_3 dissociates to **bicarbonate** (HCO$_3^-$) and H$^+$ (Fig. 10b; Chapter 9). We produce ~15 moles of CO_2 per day, corresponding to a large acid load. CO_2 easily crosses cell membranes, so also affects intracellular pH. By convention other acids are called **metabolic** or **fixed** acids because they cannot be excreted by the lungs. All acids other than H_2CO_3 are fixed, and result from incomplete oxidation of carbohydrates (e.g. lactate), protein (phosphate, sulphate) and fats (ketones). About 60 mmol of fixed acids are generated daily, just ~1% of that from CO_2 production, explaining the strong influence that ventilation has on acid–base status. Renal mechanisms are however still crucially important. The liver also contributes because it is a major source of CO_2, metabolises fixed acid anions and generates ammonium (see below). A low blood [H$^+$] can be maintained despite high levels of acid production because blood contains **buffers**, and acid is excreted by the lungs (as CO_2) and kidneys (Fig. 10b).

Buffers

Buffering is the ability of a solution to limit (but not prevent) changes in pH when acid (or alkali) is added. Acids are H$^+$ donors, and bases H$^+$ acceptors; **buffers** are mixtures of **weak acids** and their **conjugate bases**. Whilst **strong acids** dissociate completely in solution (e.g. HCL $\rightarrow$ H$^+$ + Cl$^-$), weak acids dissociate incompletely, so solutions contain both the acid and their conjugate base. When H$^+$ is added to such a solution, some combines with the conjugate base to form more weak acid (e.g. H$^+$ + HCO$_3^+$ $\rightarrow$ H$_2$CO$_3$ [$\rightarrow$ CO$_2$]), so limiting the rise in [H$^+$] (thus fall in pH). Similarly, the rise in pH on adding alkali (i.e. OH$^-$ + H$^+$ $\rightarrow$ H$_2$O) is limited by release of H$^+$ from weak acids. The pH at which [weak acid] and [conjugate base] are equal corresponds to their **pK$_A$** (negative log of dissociation constant, K$_A$), and is the point at which buffering is most effective (least change in pH per unit acid/alkali added). The relationship between pH, [weak acid] and [conjugate base] is described by the **Henderson–Hasselbalch equation** and illustrated by **buffer curves** (Figs. 10c and 10d).

The body has a very large buffering capacity. The most important buffers in blood are **bicarbonate** and **haemoglobin**; others are shown in Figure 10e. Bicarbonate is the conjugate base for H_2CO_3 (thus effectively CO_2). The [H_2CO_3] is proportional to [CO_2], which is calculated from Pco$_2$ × CO_2 solubility; thus when [HCO$_3^-$] = 24 mmol/L and Pco$_2$ = 5.3 kPa (40 mmHg), pH is 7.4 (Fig. 10c). A **key point** is that whatever their concentrations, if the ratio [HCO$_3^-$]/[CO$_2$] remains at 20 then pH will be 7.4 (i.e. log 20 × 6.1; see Fig. 11a). Although the pK$_A$ for bicarbonate buffer (6.1) is far from the pH of blood (7.4), it still acts as an effective buffer because Pco$_2$ and HCO$_3^-$ are controlled by ventilation (Chapter 11) and the kidneys (see below).

Proteins act as buffers because their amino acid residues can donate or accept H$^+$. **Haemoglobin** is particularly effective because it has large numbers of histidine residues with a pK$_A$ close to 7.4. However, this is affected by oxygenation, so the pK$_A$ for oxyhaemoglobin is 6.8, and for deoxyhaemoglobin is 7.8. This explains why deoxyhaemoglobin is the better buffer (Chapter 9). All other blood proteins combined contribute only ~20% of the buffering capacity of haemoglobin.

Control of acid–base balance

Acid–base balance can only be achieved if the rate of acid production is matched by that of excretion; accumulation of acid (or too greater loss) leads to acidosis or alkalosis (Chapter 11). Most acid is excreted as CO_2 by the lungs, and ventilation is regulated by arterial Pco$_2$ and pH (Chapter 12). As Pco$_2$ has a major influence on acid–base status, control of ventilation and acid–base balance are inextricably linked, and respiratory dysfunction has profound effects on acid–base status (Chapter 11). Altering ventilation has rapid effects on blood pH (minutes) (Fig. 10b).

The kidneys provide a slower means of acid–base regulation (hours, days), by excreting H$^+$ from fixed acids and regulating HCO$_3^-$. Intercalated cells in the distal nephron secrete H$^+$ into the lumen where they combine with urinary buffers (ammonia, phosphate) and are subsequently eliminated in the urine, which is therefore normally acid. Bicarbonate filtered by the glomerulus is normally completely reabsorbed, primarily in the proximal convoluted tubule, so none is excreted in the urine. However, in alkaline conditions bicarbonate can be excreted, and in acid conditions intercalated cells generate "new" bicarbonate from CO_2. These cells contain carbonic anhydrase, speeding the combination of CO_2 and water to produce H_2CO_3 which dissociates to H$^+$ and HCO$_3^-$. H$^+$ is excreted in the urine as above, whilst HCO$_3^-$ enters the blood.

Regulation of acid–base balance is thus provided by both lungs and kidneys (Fig. 10b), and dysfunction of either will compromise a patient's acid–base status. However, the duality of regulation and the dynamic nature of the bicarbonate buffer system means that one can **compensate** for failures in the other, by altering either [CO$_2$] or [HCO$_3^-$] such that their ratio returns towards 20, and pH towards 7.4 (see above and Chapter 11).

11 Acid–base disorders

Figure 11a Relationship between [HCO₃⁻] and $P_a\text{co}_2$ at different pH

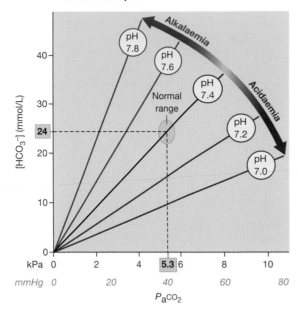

Figure 11b Davenport diagram

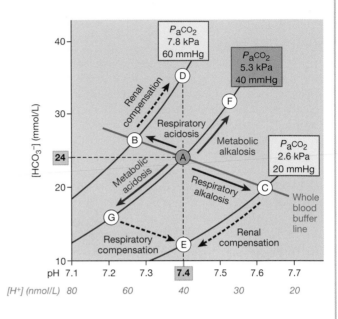

Figure 11c Types and causes of acid–base disorders and associated changes in pH and $P_a\text{co}_2$

For simple respiratory acid-base disorders, pH and $P_a\text{co}_2$ change in opposite directions; for simple metabolic disorders they change in the same direction.

	Direction of change in:			Direction of change in:	
	pH	$P_a\text{co}_2$		pH	$P_a\text{co}_2$
Respiratory acidosis *(hypoventilation)*			**Respiratory alkalosis** *(hyperventilation)*		
Respiratory failure	↓	↑	High levels of anxiety	↑	↓
Obstructive respiratory diseases			Pain		
Restrictive respiratory diseases			Hypoxia, altitude *(stimulates breathing) (... but can also cause lactic acidosis)*		
Respiratory neuromuscular disease					
Depression of respiratory centres *(e.g. head trauma, drugs)*			Excessive mechanical ventilation		
Obesity hypoventilation syndrome					
Inadequate mechanical ventilation					
Metabolic acidosis *(normal anion gap)*			**Metabolic alkalosis**		
Diarrhoea, loss of HCO₃⁻ from gut	↓	↓	Vomiting, loss of gastric acid — *Most common*	↑	↑
Renal tubular acidosis			Diuretics		
Metabolic acidosis *(high anion gap)*			Volume depletion — ↑ *Loss of acid from kidney*		
			Hypokalaemia		
Renal failure or tubular damage			Excess aldosterone		
Lactic acidosis *(hypoxia, sepsis)*			Antacid abuse		
Ketoacidosis *(e.g. diabetes, starvation)*					
Toxins *(e.g. methanol, salicylate)*					

Figure 11d Anion gap

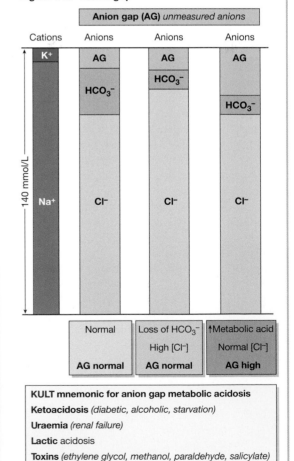

The Respiratory System at a Glance, Fourth Edition. Jeremy P.T. Ward. © Jeremy P.T. Ward. Published 2015 by John Wiley & Sons, Ltd.

Perturbations of acid–base status are common, particularly in respiratory and renal disease because of the key role the lungs and kidneys play in acid–base balance (Chapter 10). To limit confusion, one should properly use the term **acidaemia** for an arterial blood pH <7.35, and **alkalaemia** for pH >7.45 (*-aemia = of blood*). **Acidosis** and **alkalosis** are reserved to describe the underlying pathology, for example, respiratory acidosis due to respiratory failure; metabolic alkalosis due to vomiting and loss of gastric acid. This becomes important when considering **mixed** acid–base disorders with two opposing processes, for example, respiratory failure (respiratory acidosis) plus vomiting (metabolic acidosis, see below). pH alone provides little information about acid–base status. **Key point**: although acidaemia is <u>always</u> accompanied by an acidosis (its cause), an acidosis may not be accompanied by acidaemia if there is also an alkalosis (similarly for alkalaemia).

Figure 11a shows the relationship between P_{CO_2}, $[HCO_3^-]$ and pH derived from the Henderson–Hasselbalch equation (Chapter 10). The gradient ($[HCO_3^-]/P_{CO_2}$) of each radiating line determines the $[H^+]$ and so pH (see Fig. 10c); thus whatever the $[HCO_3^-]$ and P_{CO_2}, if their ratio remains constant so does pH. This illustrates how changes in P_{CO_2} can be compensated by changes in $[HCO_3^-]$, and vice versa. Figure 11b shows an alternative plot of $[HCO_3^-]$ against pH, the curved lines now indicating P_{CO_2} (*Davenport diagram*). This is a commonly used format for illustrating acid–base disorders and compensation. The line marked BAC is the **buffer line** for whole blood; if [haemoglobin] is normal (anaemia or polycythaemia alters its slope), changes in P_{CO_2} alter $[HCO_3^-]$ and pH along this line. Point A represents normal conditions: pH 7.4, $[HCO_3^-]$ 24 mmol/L, P_{CO_2} 5.3 kPa (40 mmHg).

Respiratory and metabolic disorders

Figure 11c shows conditions associated with acid–base disorders. The most common are **respiratory disease** and **hypoventilation**. Acute failure of adequate ventilation (**acute respiratory failure**) leads to a rise in P_{CO_2} (hypercapnia), thereby decreasing the ratio $[HCO_3^-]/P_{CO_2}$ and so pH. This is **respiratory acidosis**, represented in Figure 11b by the arrow from A to B. **Respiratory alkalosis** (hyperventilation) is represented by the arrow from A to C. A sustained respiratory acidosis in **chronic respiratory failure** (Chapter 25) can be partially compensated by the kidneys (**renal compensation**) over a few days through increased regeneration of HCO_3^- and excretion of H^+ (Chapter 10). The $[HCO_3^-]/P_{CO_2}$ ratio is thus partially restored and pH returns towards normal (Fig. 11b, B→D). Conversely, respiratory alkalosis can be compensated by increased renal excretion of HCO_3^- (C→E).

Metabolic acid–base disorders entail changes in $[HCO_3^-]$ rather than CO_2. **Metabolic acidosis** is characterized by a low $[HCO_3^-]$ (Fig. 11b, G), due either to loss of HCO_3^- (e.g. diarrhoea, renal tubular dysfunction), or to increased production of fixed acids, renal failure or some toxins (Fig. 11c); all the latter are associated with a **high anion gap** (see below). Metabolic acidosis can be partially compensated by increased ventilation and reduction of P_{CO_2} (Fig. 11b, G→E, **respiratory compensation**),

initiated by acid stimulation of the chemoreceptors (Chapter 12). Thus diabetic ketoacidosis is associated with Kussmaul respiration (laboured hyperventilation). **Metabolic alkalosis** (Fig. 11b, F) is most commonly caused by vomiting and loss of gastric acids, or diuretic therapy which increases urine acid loss. There is limited scope for respiratory compensation of metabolic alkalosis, as it could require unsustainable falls in ventilation.

Patients often present with **mixed** respiratory and metabolic disorders, especially if hospitalized and critically ill. Examples: a COPD patient on diuretics (respiratory acidosis plus metabolic alkalosis), or with circulatory failure (respiratory acidosis plus metabolic acidosis due to lactate from tissue hypoxia). Generally, respiratory and metabolic disorders coexist when P_{CO_2} and $[HCO_3^-]$ change in opposite directions. A basic approach to diagnosis of acid–base disorders is provided after Case study 11.

Anion gap and base excess

The **anion gap** is an artefact of measurement used to assist diagnosis of the type and severity of a metabolic acidosis. It is the difference between the total concentration of **measured** cations (Na^+, sometimes plus K^+) and of **measured** anions (Cl^- and HCO_3^-). As there is never any actual difference between total [cations] and [anions] in solution, the anion gap represents the concentration of **unmeasured** anions (e.g. proteins, organic acids, sulphate and phosphate) (Fig. 11d). The normal anion gap ($[Na^+] + [K^+]) - ([Cl^-] + [HCO_3^-])$) is about 12 mmol/L, but reference ranges differ depending on method of measurement, and whether K^+ is excluded.

$[HCO_3^-]$ is reduced in metabolic acidosis. If this is due to loss of HCO_3^- (e.g. diarrhoea, some renal conditions), HCO_3^- is replaced by Cl^- to maintain neutrality and the anion gap is normal (**hyperchloraemic** acidosis). However, if $[HCO_3^-]$ is reduced because H^+ from metabolic acids has been buffered by HCO_3^- thus forming CO_2 (e.g. lactic acidosis, diabetic ketoacidosis; Chapter 10), neutrality is maintained by their remaining anions (e.g. lactate, ketone bases) which are not measured, so the anion gap increases (Fig. 11d). Thus a high anion gap indicates production of metabolic acids (an **anion gap metabolic acidosis**). Important point: As albumin is the major unmeasured anion in plasma, **hypoalbuminaemia** reduces the anion gap, and so could mask a rise due to metabolic acids.

Base excess (or deficit) represents the excess $[HCO_3^-]$ compared to normal $[HCO_3^-]$ *if P_{CO_2} was first corrected back to 5.3 kPa (40 mmHg)*. It thus indicates whether the acid–base disturbance includes metabolic or compensatory components (i.e. excess or deficit of HCO_3^-). In a pure, *acute* respiratory acidosis correction of P_{CO_2} back to normal would by definition return pH and $[HCO_3^-]$ back to normal, so there is no base deficit. It can be calculated by blood gas analysers or by using a nomogram from the pH, P_{CO_2} and [haemoglobin] (to correct for buffering). A base deficit more than +2 or less than −2 mmol/L indicates metabolic alkalosis or acidosis respectively, or renal compensation. For example, the base excess for the fully compensated respiratory acidosis shown in Figure 11b is the difference in $[HCO_3^-]$ between points A and D (~+12 mmol/L).

12 Control of breathing I: chemical mechanisms

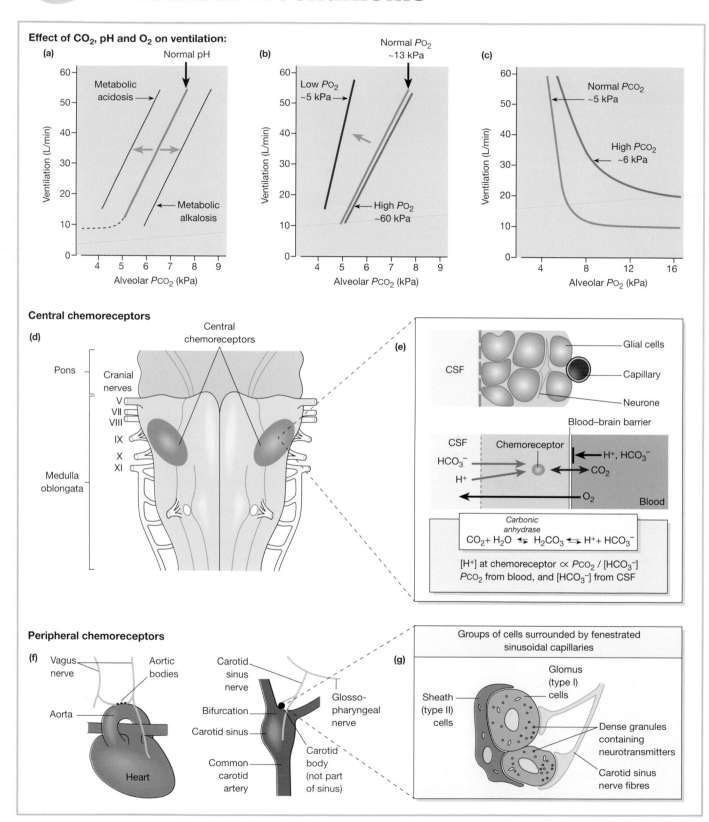

Effect of CO₂, pH and O₂ on ventilation:

(a) — Ventilation (L/min) vs Alveolar P_{CO_2} (kPa): Normal pH, Metabolic acidosis, Metabolic alkalosis

(b) — Ventilation (L/min) vs Alveolar P_{CO_2} (kPa): Normal P_{O_2} ~13 kPa, Low P_{O_2} ~5 kPa, High P_{O_2} ~60 kPa

(c) — Ventilation (L/min) vs Alveolar P_{O_2} (kPa): Normal P_{CO_2} ~5 kPa, High P_{CO_2} ~6 kPa

Central chemoreceptors

(d) Pons, Cranial nerves V, VII, VIII, IX, X, XI, Medulla oblongata, Central chemoreceptors

(e) Glial cells, CSF, Capillary, Neurone

Blood–brain barrier

CSF, Chemoreceptor, HCO_3^-, H^+, H^+, HCO_3^-, CO_2, O_2, Blood

Carbonic anhydrase
$$CO_2 + H_2O \leftrightarrows H_2CO_3 \leftrightarrows H^+ + HCO_3^-$$

$[H^+]$ at chemoreceptor $\propto P_{CO_2} / [HCO_3^-]$
P_{CO_2} from blood, and $[HCO_3^-]$ from CSF

Peripheral chemoreceptors

(f) Vagus nerve, Aortic bodies, Aorta, Heart

Carotid sinus nerve, Glosso-pharyngeal nerve, Bifurcation, Carotid sinus, Common carotid artery, Carotid body (not part of sinus)

(g) Groups of cells surrounded by fenestrated sinusoidal capillaries

Glomus (type I) cells, Sheath (type II) cells, Dense granules containing neurotransmitters, Carotid sinus nerve fibres

The Respiratory System at a Glance, Fourth Edition. Jeremy P.T. Ward. © Jeremy P.T. Ward. Published 2015 by John Wiley & Sons, Ltd.

Chemical control of ventilation is mediated via **central** and **peripheral chemoreceptors**, which detect arterial P_{CO_2} and pH (central and peripheral) and P_{O_2} (peripheral only), and modulate ventilation via a distributed network of neurones in the **brainstem** (Chapter 13). P_{CO_2} is the most important factor. The chemoreceptors allow arterial P_{CO_2} and P_{O_2} to be maintained within narrow limits despite large changes in metabolism (e.g. exercise), although ventilation in exercise is also affected by other factors (Chapter 16).

Ventilatory response to changes in P_{A,CO_2} and P_{A,O_2}

Normal alveolar P_{CO_2} ($P_{A}CO_2$) is approximately 5.3 kPa (40 mmHg). Increasing $P_{A}CO_2$ causes minute ventilation (litres ventilated per minute) to rise in an almost linear fashion (Fig. 12a), by approximately 15–25 L/min for each kPa rise in $P_{A}CO_2$ (~2.7 L/min per mmHg). There is considerable variation between individuals, and athletes and patients with chronic respiratory disease often have a reduced response to $P_{A}CO_2$ (Chapters 28 and 46). If $P_{A}CO_2$ increases above 10 kPa, ventilation decreases due to direct suppression of central respiratory neurones. **Metabolic acidosis** (an increase in [H+] caused by reduced [HCO_3^-]; see Chapter 10) shifts the CO_2–ventilation response curve to the left, whereas **metabolic alkalosis** shifts it to the right (Fig. 12a). Note that a rise in [H+] caused by increased P_{CO_2} is called **respiratory acidosis**. Increasing $P_{A}O_2$ from the normal value of approximately 13 kPa (~100 mmHg) has little effect on the CO_2–ventilation response curve, but if the $P_{A}O_2$ is reduced, the slope of the relationship becomes steeper and ventilation increases for any given rise in $P_{A}CO_2$ (Fig. 12b). When the effect of $P_{A}O_2$ is investigated independently (at constant $P_{A}CO_2$), there is little increase in ventilation until the $P_{A}O_2$ falls below approximately 8 kPa (~60 mmHg) (Fig. 12c). The effect of reducing $P_{A}O_2$ is however potentiated if the $P_{A}CO_2$ is raised – that is, there is a **synergistic** (more than additive) relationship between the effects of $P_{A}O_2$ and $P_{A}CO_2$.

The central chemoreceptor

The **central chemoreceptor** consists of a diffuse collection of neurones located near the ventrolateral surface of the medulla, close to the exit of IX and X cranial nerves (and probably elsewhere) (Fig. 12d). These are sensitive to the pH of the surrounding cerebrospinal fluid (CSF) and do **not** respond to P_{O_2}. CSF is separated from blood by the **blood–brain barrier**, a tight endothelial layer lining the blood vessels of the brain. This barrier is impermeable to polar (charged) molecules such as H+ and HCO_3^-, but CO_2 can diffuse across it easily. The pH of CSF is therefore determined by the arterial P_{CO_2} and the CSF [HCO_3^-] (Chapter 10), and is not directly affected by changes in blood pH (Fig. 12e). CSF contains little protein, so its buffering capacity is low; therefore, a small change in P_{CO_2} will cause a large change in CSF pH. Stimulation of the central chemoreceptor by a fall in CSF pH (rise in blood P_{CO_2}) causes an increase in ventilation. The central chemoreceptor is thought to be responsible for approximately 80% of the response to CO_2 in humans.

It has a relatively slow response time (~20 seconds), as CO_2 has to diffuse across the blood–brain barrier.

The peripheral chemoreceptors

The **peripheral chemoreceptors** are within the **carotid** and **aortic bodies**. The carotid body is a small (~2 mg) structure located at the bifurcation of the common carotid artery, just above the carotid sinus. It is innervated by the carotid sinus nerve, leading to the glossopharyngeal (Fig. 12f). The aortic bodies are distributed around the aortic arch and are innervated by the vagus. In humans, they are much less important than carotid bodies. The carotid body contains **glomus** (type I) cells and **sheath** (type II) cells (Fig. 12g). Glomus cells are responsible for chemoreception; they have dense granules containing neurotransmitters and contact axons of the carotid sinus nerve. The function of sheath cells may be to protect and support the glomus cells, analogous to glial cells in the central nervous system.

Carotid bodies respond to increased P_{CO_2} or [H+] and decreased P_{O_2} (**not** blood O_2 content) by increasing firing rate in the carotid sinus nerve, and thus ventilation. They have a high blood flow and consequently a small arteriovenous difference for P_{CO_2} and P_{O_2}. They respond rapidly (seconds) and are sufficiently fast to detect small oscillations in blood gases associated with breathing. The mechanisms by which changes in P_{CO_2}, pH and P_{O_2} are detected are not fully understood, but are believed to involve inhibition of K+ channels in the glomus cell, with consequent depolarization, Ca^{2+} entry and release of neurotransmitters in the dense granules.

Adaptation: chronic respiratory disease and altitude

When hypercapnia (raised arterial P_{CO_2}) is prolonged, for example in chronic respiratory disease, CSF pH gradually returns to normal due to an adaptive and compensatory increase in HCO_3^- transport across the blood–brain barrier. Similarly, renal compensation of the associated respiratory acidosis (Chapter 11) returns the pH of the blood towards normal, so reducing stimulation of the peripheral chemoreceptors by the acidosis. The drive to breathe from the central and peripheral chemoreceptors are consequently reduced, even though P_{CO_2} is still high. Associated with this, there is occasionally a loss of sensitivity to further increases in $P_{a}CO_2$, and the patient's ventilation is then primarily controlled by the level of $P_{a}O_2$ (**hypoxic drive**). Care must be taken with such patients, as giving high concentrations of O_2 in order to increase blood O_2 saturation may raise the $P_{a}O_2$ sufficiently to depress the hypoxic drive and hence ventilation. Normally, approximately 23–28% O_2 is given to such patients. This leads to a sufficiently small rise in $P_{a}O_2$ as to have little effect on the hypoxic drive, but because of the steep slope of the O_2 dissociation curve (Chapter 8), it can result in a significant improvement in O_2 content.

At high altitudes, ventilation is stimulated by the low atmospheric P_{O_2}. This leads to **hypocapnia** and alkalosis (as more CO_2 is blown off), which depress ventilation. Over some days, the pH of CSF returns to normal due to HCO_3^- transport out of the CSF, even though the P_{CO_2} remains low, and consequently ventilation increases again. Blood pH also returns towards normal due to renal compensation (Chapter 11), similarly reducing alkalosis-induced depression of the peripheral chemoreceptors. These processes form part of the **acclimatization to altitude**.

13 Control of breathing II: neural mechanisms

Figure 13 Neural pathways

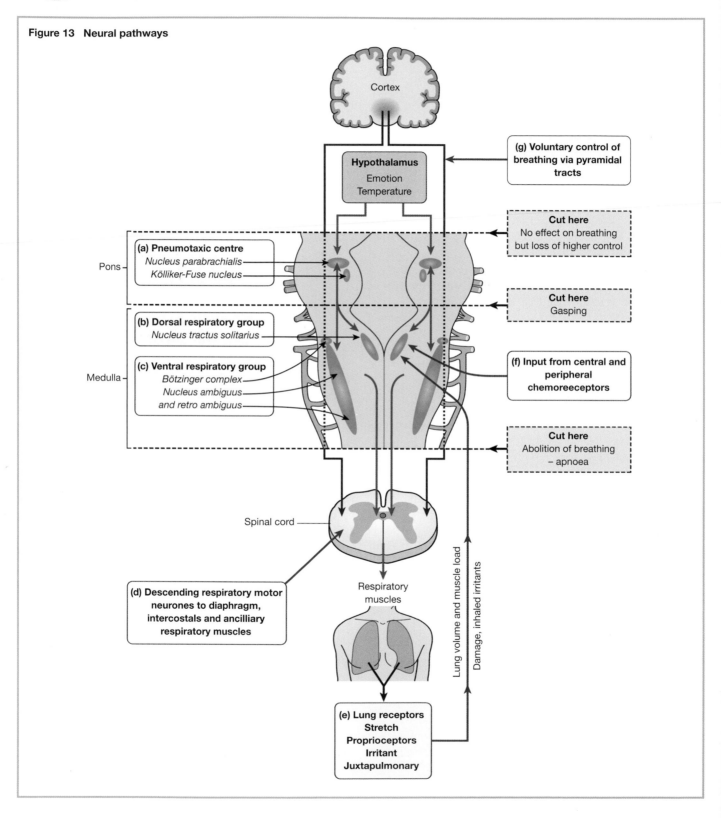

Control of breathing involves a **central pattern generator** in the brainstem that sets the basic rhythm and pattern of ventilation and controls the respiratory muscles. It is modulated by higher centres and feedback from **sensors**, including **chemoreceptors** (Chapter 12) and lung **mechanoreceptors**. The neural networks involved are complex, reflecting the need to coordinate ventilation with functions such as coughing, swallowing and vocalization.

Brainstem and central pattern generator

The **central pattern generator** determines the rate and pattern of breathing, and is a complex network encompassing diffuse groups of respiratory neurones in the **pons** and **medulla**. These contain **inspiratory** and **expiratory** neurones, with activity corresponding to inspiration and expiration, although others show more complex relationships. **Reciprocal inhibition** means activity of inspiratory neurones inhibits activity of expiratory neurones, and vice versa.

The **medulla** contains two groups of respiratory neurones. The **dorsal respiratory group** (DRG; Fig. 13b) in the **nucleus tractus solitarii** contains inspiratory neurones and receives ascending input from central and peripheral chemoreceptors (Chapter 12; Fig. 13f), and from lung receptors via the vagus (Fig. 13e). The ventrolateral medulla contains a column of neurones extending from the lateral reticular nucleus and through the **nucleus ambiguus**, comprising the **caudal** (expiratory neurones) and **rostral** (inspiratory neurones) **ventral respiratory groups** (VRG) and **pre-Bötzinger** and **Bötzinger** complexes (Fig. 13c). Although the pre-Bötzinger complex contains neurones with intrinsic activity (pacemakers), these may only be associated with **gasping**, an autoresuscitative mechanism following hypoxia, as sectioning between the medulla and pons tends to abolish eupnoea (normal breathing) and lead to gasping in the absence of vagal input. Descending output from the medulla regulates activity of respiratory muscle motor neurones (intercostals, phrenic (diaphragm), abdominal) (Fig. 13d).

The **pneumotaxic centre** is located in the **nucleus parabrachialis** and **Kölliker–Fuse nucleus** of the **pons** (Fig. 13a), and has a critical role in eupnoea and mediating responses to lung receptor stimulation (see below). It receives ascending input from the VRG, although vagal input from lung stretch receptors is routed via the DRG. The input from stretch receptors is important for timing of respiratory rhythm and especially switching inspiration off as lung volume increases. In the absence of vagal input, sectioning the mid-pons causes **apneusis** (prolonged inspiratory effort with short expirations); it has therefore been suggested that there is an **apneustic centre** in the caudal pons, possibly associated with the Kölliker–Fuse nucleus. Descending input from the hypothalamus and higher centres mediates the effects of factors such as emotion and temperature on breathing, but eupnoea is maintained following sectioning above the pons (Fig. 13), although voluntary control is lost. Voluntary control of breathing is mediated by motor neurones from the cortex contained in the **pyramidal tracts**, which bypass the pneumotaxic and medullary respiratory areas (Fig. 13g). Certain rare brainstem lesions can leave the voluntary pathways intact while impairing brainstem mechanisms, so ventilation may cease when the patient falls asleep (*Ondine's curse*; Chapter 46).

The **origin of the respiratory rhythm** is controversial. Whereas some place this in the VRG and pre-Bötzinger complex, others suggest a *switching concept*, with eupnoea reflecting the output of a pontomedullary neuronal circuit that includes pneumotaxic (and apneustic) centres, VRG and DRG. In either case, cycling or switching due to reciprocal inhibition and 'off switches' within these networks is probably the source of the rhythm of breathing rather than specific pacemaker neurones.

Lung receptors and reflexes

Stretch receptors are located in the smooth muscle of the bronchial walls. These are mostly **slowly adapting** (continue to fire with sustained stimulation). Their afferent nerves ascend via the vagus. Stimulation of stretch receptors causes inspiration to be shorter and shallower and delays the next cycle. These receptors are largely responsible for the **Hering–Breuer inspiratory reflex**, where lung inflation inhibits inspiratory muscle activity. Conversely, the **deflation reflex** augments inspiratory muscle activity on lung deflation. These reflexes are weak during normal breathing in adults, but become more relevant when tidal volume is large (>1 L, e.g. in exercise). The reflex is very sensitive in neonates to protect the lungs against overinflation due to the highly compliant nature of the chest wall.

Juxtapulmonary or 'J' receptors are located on alveolar and bronchial walls, close to the capillaries. Their afferents are small unmyelinated (C-fibre) or myelinated nerves in the vagus. Activation causes **apnoea** (cessation of breathing) or rapid shallow breathing, falls in heart rate and blood pressure, laryngeal constriction and relaxation of skeletal muscles. J receptors are stimulated by increased alveolar wall fluid, pulmonary congestion and oedema, microembolisms and inflammatory mediators such as histamine – all of which are associated with lung disease. The general action of J receptors is depression of somatic and visceral activity, which may be appropriate for serious lung damage as this would suppress metabolism in the face of compromised gas exchange.

Irritant receptors are located throughout airways between epithelial cells, with rapidly adapting afferent myelinated fibres in the vagus. Receptors in the trachea lead to cough – those in lower airways to hyperpnoea. They also cause reflex bronchial and laryngeal constrictions. Irritant receptors are stimulated by irritant gases, smoke and dust (Chapters 19 and 35), but also by rapid large inflations and deflations, airway deformation, pulmonary congestion and inflammation. Irritant receptors are responsible for the deep augmented breaths or sighs seen every 5–20 minutes at rest, which reverse the slow collapse of the lungs that occurs in quiet breathing. They may be involved with the first deep gasps of the newborn ('first breath') and the Hering–Breuer deflationary reflex.

Proprioceptors (position/length sensors) are located in the Golgi tendon organs, muscle spindles and joints of the respiratory muscles, but not diaphragm. Afferents lead to the spinal cord via dorsal roots, stimulated by shortening and load in respiratory muscles, although not diaphragm. They are important for coping with increased load and achieving optimal tidal volume and frequency. Input from non-respiratory muscles and joints can also stimulate breathing, for example, during exercise.

Other receptors that may modulate respiration

Pain receptors: stimulation often causes brief apnoea followed by increased breathing.

Receptors in the *trigeminal region* and *larynx*: stimulation may give rise to apnoea or laryngeal spasm.

Arterial baroreceptors: increases in blood pressure, particularly if rapid, may depress breathing (and vice versa); reason not fully understood.

14 Pulmonary circulation and anatomical right-to-left shunts

Figure 14a Pulmonary and systemic circulation and normal anatomical right-to-left shunts

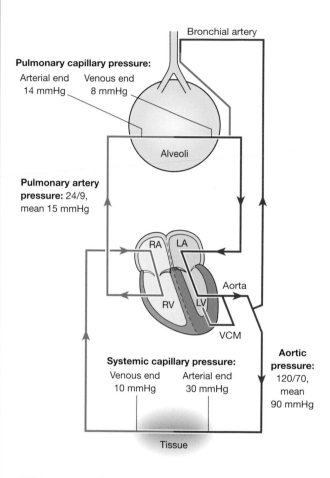

Bronchial artery

Pulmonary capillary pressure:
Arterial end   Venous end
14 mmHg   8 mmHg

Alveoli

Pulmonary artery pressure: 24/9, mean 15 mmHg

RA   LA

Aorta

RV   LV

VCM

Systemic capillary pressure:
Venous end   Arterial end
10 mmHg   30 mmHg

Aortic pressure: 120/70, mean 90 mmHg

Tissue

VCM = venae cordis minimae (Thebesian veins)

Figure 14b The initial effects of a 20% right-to-left shunt on arterial O_2 and CO_2 contents and partial pressures

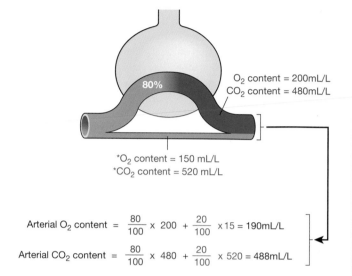

80%

O_2 content = 200mL/L
CO_2 content = 480mL/L

*O_2 content = 150 mL/L
*CO_2 content = 520 mL/L

$$\text{Arterial } O_2 \text{ content} = \frac{80}{100} \times 200 + \frac{20}{100} \times 15 = 190\text{mL/L}$$

$$\text{Arterial } CO_2 \text{ content} = \frac{80}{100} \times 480 + \frac{20}{100} \times 520 = 488\text{mL/L}$$

*Note: The mixed venous contents used are normal values. In fact, the abnormal arterial contents would lead to abnormal mixed venous contents so this simple analysis underestimates the final effect on arterial contents.

The P_{O_2} and P_{CO_2} that result from these O_2 and CO_2 contents can be found from the O_2 and CO_2 dissociation curves:

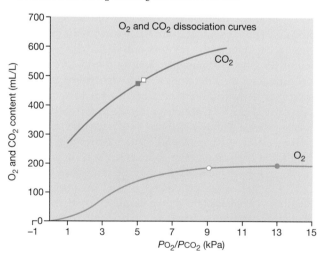

●■ Normal arterial O_2 and CO_2 pressures and contents

○□ Arterial O_2 and CO_2 pressures and contents following mixing 20% mixed venous blood with 80% blood undergoing normal gas exchange

O_2 and CO_2 dissociation curves

CO_2

O_2

O_2 and CO_2 content (mL/L)

P_{O_2}/P_{CO_2} (kPa)

The Respiratory System at a Glance, Fourth Edition. Jeremy P.T. Ward. © Jeremy P.T. Ward. Published 2015 by John Wiley & Sons, Ltd.

Pulmonary circulation compared with the systemic circulation

The **pulmonary circulation** is in series with the **systemic circulation**, and pulmonary blood flow nearly equals aortic blood flow (Fig. 14a). **Pulmonary vascular resistance** is only about one-sixth of systemic resistance, and the thin-walled right ventricle need only generate a mean **pulmonary artery pressure** of about 15 mmHg to drive the cardiac output through the lungs. Systemic pressures are higher (Fig. 14a), dropping steeply across the main resistance vessels, the arterioles, to give a capillary flow that is usually non-pulsatile. Pulmonary vascular resistance is more evenly distributed in the microcirculation and pulmonary capillary flow remains pulsatile.

Local systemic resistance and blood flow are controlled by sympathetic nerves, metabolites and other substances acting on arterioles. Both sympathetic and parasympathetic nerves innervate pulmonary vessels, but their influence is weak in most circumstances. Systemic arterioles dilate in response to hypoxia, increasing flow and hence oxygen delivery to hypoxic tissues. In contrast, **hypoxic pulmonary vasoconstriction** occurs in the pulmonary circulation. This response, which is accentuated by high P_{CO_2}, improves gas exchange by diverting blood from underventilated to well-ventilated regions (Chapter 15). The response is unhelpful in the presence of global lung hypoxia, at altitude or in respiratory failure, where it may contribute to the development of pulmonary hypertension and right-sided heart failure.

Systemic vascular beds (especially the renal and cerebral) respond to changes in perfusion pressure by constricting or dilating to hold blood flow fairly constant. This **autoregulation** does not occur in the pulmonary circulation. As venous return increases in exercise, pulmonary vascular resistance falls as vessels are recruited and distended, pulmonary blood flow increases and the rise in pulmonary arterial pressure is small. The pulmonary circulation acts as a blood reservoir and the volume it contains varies, being about 450 mL when upright and 800 mL when lying down. Inspiration also increases pulmonary vascular volume.

Fluid balance across capillaries is determined by hydrostatic and oncotic pressures (the **Starling forces**; see *The Cardiovascular System at a Glance*) across capillary walls. **Capillary oncotic pressure** opposes filtration and is about 27 mmHg in both circulations. Although hydrostatic pressure is low in the pulmonary capillaries (~10 mmHg), net filtration of fluid occurs in pulmonary capillaries as it does in systemic capillaries. Other factors favouring filtration are **interstitial oncotic pressure**, which is relatively high in the lungs (about 18 mmHg) and **interstitial hydrostatic pressure**, which is negative (about −4 mmHg). **Pulmonary oedema** occurs when these forces are altered to increase net filtration above the rate that can be cleared by the pulmonary lymphatics. For example, it may occur when pulmonary capillary pressure is increased in **mitral stenosis** and **left ventricular failure**. **Inspiratory crepitations** (crackles) on auscultation in these conditions are probably caused by popping open of airways in lungs stiffened by congestion with blood. They are most obvious at the bases, where hydrostatic pressure is highest. Pulmonary congestion and oedema (and hence breathlessness in these conditions) are worsened by the increase in pulmonary blood volume lying down.

Anatomical or true right-to-left shunts

Ideally, all venous blood emerging from tissues would return to the right side of the heart to be pumped through the gas-exchanging lung. In fact, part of the blood draining the **bronchial circulation** joins the pulmonary vein. This part results in deoxygenated blood from the airways contaminating blood returning from alveoli (Fig. 14a). In addition, a small amount of the coronary venous blood drains directly into the left ventricular cavity via the **venae cordis minimae (Thebesian veins)**. These additions of deoxygenated (right-sided) blood to oxygenated (left-sided) blood are known as anatomical **right-to-left shunts**. In healthy people, they are equivalent to 2% or less of the cardiac output, but they explain why arterial P_{O_2} is less than alveolar P_{O_2} even though pulmonary capillary blood equilibrates with alveolar gas.

In disease, right-to-left shunting of blood may be much larger. **Atelectasis** (airless lung) or **consolidation** in **pneumonia** will result in pulmonary arterial blood supplying the affected region failing to undergo gas exchange. Right-to-left shunts are also the cause of reduced arterial oxygenation in **cyanotic congenital heart disease** such as **tetralogy of Fallot**. Atrial or ventricular septal defects do not usually cause impaired gas exchange and cyanosis, as the higher left-sided pressures give rise to **left-to-right shunts** in which some oxygenated blood is pumped again through the lungs. If a large left-to-right shunt remains untreated, eventually the excessive pulmonary blood flow leads to pulmonary hypertension. As right ventricular pressure increases, the shunt through the atrial or ventricular septal defect may then reverse to give a right-to-left shunt and cyanosis (Eisenmenger's syndrome).

Effect of right-to-left shunts on arterial blood gases

In the right-to-left shunt, shown schematically in Figure 14b, 20% of blood fails to pass through functioning alveoli and its O_2 and CO_2 contents remain at mixed venous levels of 150 and 520 mL/L, respectively. Eighty per cent of the blood undergoes normal gas exchange, emerging with normal O_2 and CO_2 contents of 200 and 480 mL/L, respectively. The initial effect on arterial gas contents is calculated from a weighted average of the contents in these two bloodstreams. This gives an arterial O_2 content 10 mL/L below normal and CO_2 content 8 mL/L above normal. The effect of these changes in O_2 and CO_2 content on arterial P_{O_2} and P_{CO_2} can be determined from the relevant dissociation curve. As the O_2 dissociation curve is flat in this region there is quite a large fall in arterial P_{CO_2} to about 9 kPa (68 mmHg) compared with the normal 13 kPa (97 mmHg). The much steeper CO_2 dissociation curve means the rise in P_{CO_2} is small, from the normal value of 5.3 kPa (40 mmHg) to about 5.5 kPa (41 mmHg).

If the respiratory system is otherwise normal, the reduced P_aO_2 and increased P_aCO_2 simulate ventilation via the chemoreceptors and the CO_2 washed out of the functioning areas restores arterial CO_2 content and P_aCO_2 to normal. In contrast, increased ventilation has little effect on arterial oxygen content and P_{O_2}, as the blood draining the ventilated areas of the lung was already saturated. If hypoxia is severe, the stimulation in ventilation is often great enough to reduce P_aCO_2 below normal. Typically, in a right-to-left shunt, there is a low P_aO_2 with a normal or low P_aCO_2.

15 Ventilation–perfusion mismatching

Figure 15a Different types of V_A/Q regions

Normal	Dead space	Dead-space effect	Shunt effect	True/anatomical shunt
$\dot{V}_A$ = Normal	$\dot{V}_A$ = Normal	$\dot{V}_A$ = Normal	$\dot{V}_A$ = Low	$\dot{V}_A$ = 0
$\dot{Q}$ = Normal	$\dot{Q}$ = 0	$\dot{Q}$ = Low	$\dot{Q}$ = Normal	$\dot{Q}$ = Normal
V_A/Q = Normal (close to 1)	V_A/Q = ∞	V_A/Q = High	V_A/Q = Low	V_A/Q = 0

Figure 15b Variation of ventilation, $\dot{V}_A$, perfusion, $\dot{Q}$ and ventilation–perfusion ratio, V_A/Q with vertical height in the the upright lung

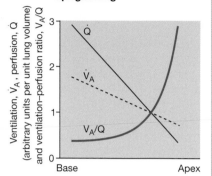

PO_2 and O_2 contents of blood from these regions breathing air and oxygen

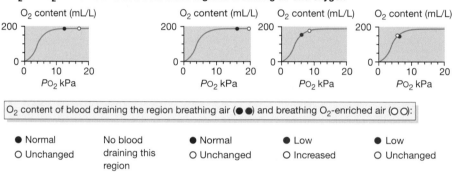

O_2 content of blood draining the region breathing air (● ●) and breathing O_2-enriched air (O O):

● Normal	No blood draining this region	● Normal	● Low	● Low
O Unchanged		O Unchanged	O Increased	O Unchanged

Alveoli at start — and end ···· of breath at different heights   Blood vessels at different heights

Figure 15c The effect of a mixture of high and low V_A/Q regions on arterial blood gases

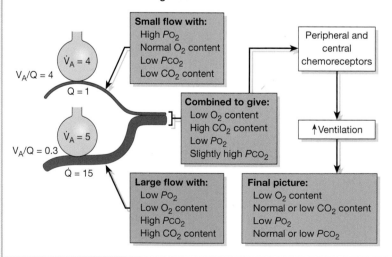

Small flow with:
High PO_2
Normal O_2 content
Low PCO_2
Low CO_2 content

Combined to give:
Low O_2 content
High CO_2 content
Low PO_2
Slightly high PCO_2

Large flow with:
Low PO_2
Low O_2 content
High PCO_2
High CO_2 content

Peripheral and central chemoreceptors

↑Ventilation

Final picture:
Low O_2 content
Normal or low CO_2 content
Low PO_2
Normal or low PCO_2

Figure 15d Alveolar air equation

This predicts the PO_2 in the functioning or 'ideal' alveoli

$$P_AO_2 \cong PIO_2 - \frac{P_aCO_2}{R}$$

$$R = \text{The respiratory gas exchange ratio} = \frac{CO_2 \text{ production}}{O_2 \text{ consumption}}$$

(R is usually about 0.8)

PIO_2 = Inspired O_2 partial pressure
P_aCO_2 = Arterial CO_2 partial pressure (≈ ideal alveolar PCO_2)

The Respiratory System at a Glance, Fourth Edition. Jeremy P.T. Ward. © Jeremy P.T. Ward. Published 2015 by John Wiley & Sons, Ltd.

At rest, alveolar ventilation and pulmonary blood flow are similar, each being around 5 L/min. Ventilation ($\dot{V}_A$) and perfusion ($\dot{Q}$) may vary in different lung regions, but for optimal gas exchange they must be matched. Areas with high perfusion need high ventilation, and, ideally, local ventilation–perfusion ratios (V_A/Q) should be close to 1. Ventilation–perfusion mismatching or inequality is said to occur when regional V_A/Q ratios vary, with many being much greater or less than 1 (Fig. 15a). A right-to-left shunt from complete collapse or consolidation of a region (Chapter 14) has $V_A/Q = 0$, and can be viewed as an extreme example of ventilation–perfusion mismatching. At the other extreme, alveolar dead space from a pulmonary embolus is a ventilated region without perfusion and $V_A/Q = \infty$. Regions where V_A/Q is much greater than 1 have excessive ventilation or **dead-space effect** and blood from them has a high Po_2 and a low Pco_2. Regions with V_A/Q much less than 1 behave qualitatively like shunts and are sources of **shunt effect** or **venous admixture**. Blood draining them has undergone some gas exchange, but Po_2 is lower and Pco_2 higher than normal. The effect on Po_2 and O_2 content draining different V_A/Q regions both during air breathing and during oxygen breathing is shown in Figure 15a (lower panel).

Effect of the upright posture on perfusion, ventilation and V_A/Q

Hydrostatic pressure in all vessels varies with vertical height above or below the heart because of the weight of blood (Fig. 15b). On standing, the increased pressure at the lung bases distends vessels, increasing flow. Pressures generated by the right side of the heart are low, and higher up the lung vascular pressures in diastole may fall below alveolar pressure at the venous end of the pulmonary capillary. In such regions, flow is reduced and determined by the difference between arterial and alveolar pressure. There may be regions at the apices, especially in haemorrhage or positive-pressure ventilation, where alveolar pressure also exceeds pressure at the arterial end of the pulmonary capillaries. The vessels collapse completely for part of each cardiac cycle, giving low intermittent flow. The net result is a blood flow per unit volume of lung tissue that falls progressively from base to apex.

Gravity also affects intrapleural pressure, which is less negative at the base than at the apex. As a result, at functional residual capacity, apical alveoli are more expanded, with less capacity for further expansion during inspiration, than at the bases. Consequently, ventilation is also higher at the base than at the apex. The effect of gravity on ventilation is less marked than on perfusion and so V_A/Q is higher at the apex than at the base. In young people, the degree of mismatching is modest and has little effect on blood gases because the regions with low V_A/Q are still ventilated enough to give a high enough Po_2 to nearly saturate the blood passing through them with oxygen. The scatter of ventilation–perfusion ratios increases with age and contributes to the reduction in P_ao_2 seen in the elderly.

Ventilation–perfusion matching in disease

Increased ventilation–perfusion mismatching is an important cause of gas exchange problems in many respiratory diseases, including asthma, chronic obstructive pulmonary disease (COPD), pneumonia and pulmonary oedema. Regions of low V_A/Q may arise when airways are partly blocked by bronchoconstriction, inflammation or secretions and high V_A/Q areas arise when pulmonary emboli are partially blocking blood flow or in emphysematous areas where capillaries are lost. **Hypoxic vasoconstriction** (Chapter 14) helps reduce the severity of ventilation–perfusion mismatching by diverting blood from regions with low V_A/Q to regions that are better ventilated.

Effect of ventilation–perfusion mismatching on arterial blood gases

Blood emerging from areas with high V_A/Q might be expected to compensate for blood from areas with low V_A/Q. This is not the case, for two reasons (Fig. 15c). First, although Po_2 will be increased in high V_A/Q regions, oxygen content is raised little, as blood is normally nearly saturated. Blood draining regions with low V_A/Q will have a low Po_2 and a significantly reduced oxygen content, especially if $Po_2 <8$ kPa, 60 mmHg. In addition, these areas contribute more blood than areas with high V_A/Q, which are typically caused by reduced perfusion. The net effect of mixing blood from areas with a wide range of ventilation–perfusion ratios is a low arterial O_2 content and P_ao_2. CO_2 content is less severely affected because the overventilated areas do lose extra CO_2 and partly compensate for low V_A/Q regions. Moreover, any abnormalities of P_ao_2 and P_aco_2 will lead to a reflex increase in ventilation, which usually corrects or overcorrects the raised P_aco_2 while being less effective at raising P_ao_2. The final arterial blood gas picture, a low P_ao_2 and a normal or low P_aco_2, is similar to that resulting from anatomical right-to-left shunts (Chapter 14).

One difference is that arterial hypoxia caused by ventilation–perfusion mismatching improves much more with oxygen therapy than that caused by a shunt. In a hypoxic patient with a pure shunt, the **oxygen-enriched air** fails to reach the shunted blood. In V_A/Q mismatching, increased oxygen fraction can increase local Po_2 in areas of low V_A/Q (Fig. 15a), giving rise to significant improvement in arterial oxygen content and pressure.

Assessment of ventilation–perfusion mismatching

Regional ventilation and perfusion can be visualized by inhalation and infusion of appropriate radioisotopes (Chapter 23). A simple but useful index of the degree of mismatching is the difference between Po_2 in gas-exchanging or 'ideal' alveoli and in arterial blood. Ideal alveolar Po_2 can be calculated from the **alveolar air equation** (Fig. 15d). An increased **A–a Po_2 gradient** (A = alveolar Po_2, a = arterial Po_2) is usually caused by ventilation–perfusion mismatching or anatomical right-to-left shunts. In healthy young people, there is a small A–a gradient (<2 kPa) arising from the normal anatomical right-to-left shunts, discussed in Chapter 14. The normal value for A–a gradient increases with age and in a healthy 80-year-old may be as high as 5 kPa (38 mmHg).

16 Exercise, altitude and diving

Table 1 Typical values in a healthy but sedentary 20-year-old man at rest and in max. exercise

	Rest	Maximal exercise
Heart rate (bpm)	70	200
Stroke volume (mL)	75	90
Cardiac output (mL/min)	5250	18 000
Arterial–mixed venous O_2 content* (mL/mL)	0.048	0.167
O_2 consumption (mL/min)	250	3000
Ventilation (mL/min)	7500	140 000
Respiratory frequency (breaths/min)	15	56
Tidal volume (mL)	500	2500

(*= O_2 extraction)

Figure 16b Typical alveolar ventilation, P_{CO_2} and P_{O_2}, at altitudes between sea level (0 m) and 6000 m for subjects exposed acutely (red solid line) and chronically (blue solid line) following acclimatization. The dashed line shows the values that would have occurred if alveolar ventilation remained at its sea level value.

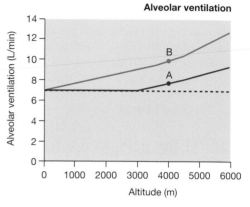

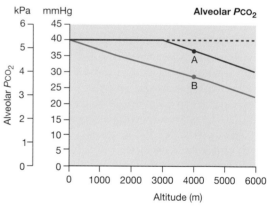

Figure 16a Typical changes in ventilation $\dot{V}$, arterial P_{O_2} (P_aO_2), arterial P_{CO_2} (P_aCO_2), arterial pH (pHa), mixed venous P_{O_2} ($P_{\bar{v}}O_2$) and mixed venous P_{CO_2} ($P_{\bar{v}}CO_2$) in a fit young man as oxygen consumption is increased from its resting value of 0.25 L/min to his maximum oxygen consumption of 4 L/min.

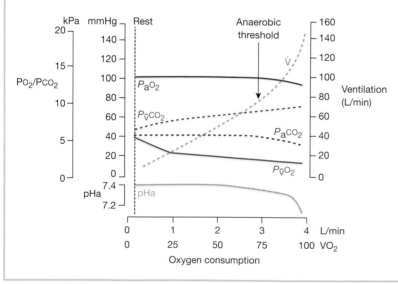

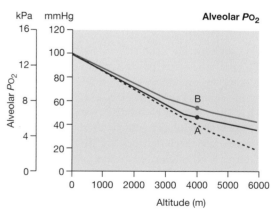

The Respiratory System at a Glance, Fourth Edition. Jeremy P.T. Ward. © Jeremy P.T. Ward. Published 2015 by John Wiley & Sons, Ltd.

Exercise

Resting arterial oxygen saturation is close to 100% and oxygen content cannot be raised significantly during exercise. **Oxygen delivery** (arterial oxygen content × blood flow) to exercising muscle is increased by increasing muscle blood flow, made possible by metabolic vasodilatation. **Oxygen extraction** from the delivered blood is also increased.

For the whole body, **oxygen consumption** (mL/min) = cardiac output (mL/min) × (arterial–mixed venous oxygen content) (mL/mL). In active muscle, oxygen unloading from haemoglobin is aided by the reduced tissue P_{O_2} and the rightward shift of the oxyhaemoglobin dissociation curve caused by local increases in P_{CO_2}, $[H^+]$ and temperature. Maximum oxygen extraction does not vary greatly with fitness, and the main factor determining **maximum oxygen consumption ($\dot{V}_{O_2}$ max)** is the maximum cardiac output. $\dot{V}_{O_2}$ max is an index of fitness and in a young man this might be 12 times resting oxygen consumption (Table 16) and more in an athlete.

In exercise, mixed venous blood has a reduced P_{O_2} and increased P_{CO_2}. As blood passes through the pulmonary capillaries, the increased alveolar to blood partial pressure gradients increase O_2 uptake and CO_2 output. In mild to moderate exercise, alveolar ventilation is accurately matched to metabolism and $P_{a}O_2$, $P_{a}CO_2$ and arterial pH (pHa) are maintained at resting values (Fig. 16a). The mechanisms initiating and controlling the ventilatory response remain uncertain. In heavy exercise, increased anaerobic metabolism increases lactic acid production and reduces arterial pH. This gives an extra stimulus to breathing via the peripheral chemoreceptors, and at this **anaerobic threshold** the relationship between ventilation and oxygen consumption becomes steeper and $P_{a}CO_2$ falls (Fig. 16a).

Exercise intolerance is a common symptom of many diseases, and the inability to raise the cardiac output adequately is the main underlying mechanism in many diseases. In anaemia oxygen delivery to the muscles is reduced because of reduced arterial oxygen content. In some respiratory diseases, limited ability to increase ventilation or incomplete equilibrium in the pulmonary capillary may limit exercise.

Altitude

Barometric pressure falls progressively with increasing altitude from about 101 kPa (760 mmHg) at sea level to 33.6 kPa (252 mmHg) on the summit of Everest (see Chapter 4), but oxygen fraction remains constant at 0.209. Moist inspired P_{O_2} ($0.209 \times (P_B - P_{H_2O})$) is about 19.9 kPa (149 mmHg) at sea level and about 5.7 kPa (43 mmHg) on the summit of Everest.

If ventilation remains unchanged, reduced inspired P_{O_2} inevitably leads to reduced $P_{a}O_2$ but $P_{a}CO_2$ ($\propto CO_2$ production/ alveolar ventilation) will be unaltered. This is the situation initially when a person ascends to altitudes up to about 3000 m (9840 ft) (Fig. 16b). Hypoxic carotid body chemoreceptor stimulation occurs, but any ventilatory increase lowers $P_{a}CO_2$, which depresses ventilation. Above 3000 m the more severe hypoxia does increase ventilation and $P_{a}CO_2$ falls (Fig. 16b). **Acute mountain sickness** commonly develops some hours after rapid ascent to altitudes above 3600 m (12,000 ft) with symptoms such as fatigue, nausea, anorexia, dizziness, headaches and sleep disturbance. It can progress to life-threatening **high-altitude pulmonary oedema** and/or **high-altitude cerebral oedema**, which usually require immediate descent. The more benign symptoms improve with time, a process known as **acclimatization**. Over the next few days, ventilation increases, raising $P_{a}O_2$ and lowering $P_{a}CO_2$ (A to B, Fig. 16b). During this period the initial alkalosis of arterial blood and cerebrospinal fluid (CSF) is corrected by bicarbonate transport out of the CSF and renal bicarbonate excretion. A gradual normalization of arterial and CSF pH was originally thought to explain the gradual increase of ventilation, but other mechanisms, such as increased sensitivity of the peripheral chemoreceptors to hypoxia and changes in the central nervous system reflex pathways, are also important. **Erythropoietin** production by the kidney is stimulated by hypoxia, and haemoglobin concentration rises from 150 g/L to around 200 g/L after a few weeks at high altitude, aiding acclimatization by increasing arterial oxygen content.

At altitude, the concentration of **2,3-diphosphoglycerate** in red blood cells increases and $P_{a}CO_2$ falls, and they cause opposite shifts (right and left respectively) of the oxyhaemoglobin dissociation curve, which at many altitudes results in little net change in oxygen affinity. At very high altitude the very low $P_{a}CO_2$ shifts the curve to the left and the beneficial effect of increased oxygen binding in the lungs outweighs the impaired oxygen release in the tissues.

With acclimatization humans can live at much higher altitudes than it is possible to tolerate acutely. The highest long-term human settlement was Quilcha, Chile (5334 m, 17,500 ft), from where miners walked to work at the Aucanquilcha mine 610 m (2000 ft) higher. Sudden exposure to the summit of Everest would cause a healthy sea level dweller to lose consciousness in less than 2 minutes but a few very fit and fully acclimatized people have climbed it without supplementary oxygen.

The hypoxic pulmonary vasoconstriction that aids ventilation–perfusion matching at sea level causes an unhelpful global vasoconstriction at high altitude. In some people living above 2500 m (8200 ft) this becomes excessive, leading to pulmonary hypertension and right ventricular failure. Excessive polycythaemia also often occurs in these patients, contributing to this **chronic mountain sickness (Monge's disease)**.

Diving

Diving into water affects the respiratory system in many ways. Breath-hold diving initiates several reflexes, leading to the cardiovascular and respiratory effects of the **diving response**. Immersion of the face in water stimulates receptors around the eyes and nose supplied by the trigeminal nerves, leading to reflex apnoea, bradycardia and widespread vasoconstriction. The apnoea helps prevent water inhalation. The oxygen-conserving bradycardia and vasoconstriction are enhanced by reflexes from the carotid body chemoreceptors but antagonized by reflexes from lung stretch receptors. The cardiovascular responses are usually modest in humans, but excessive bradycardia sometimes occurs, especially following unexpected immersion during expiration, and this may explain some accidental deaths in water.

The weight of the water increases the pressure on the body by 1 atmosphere (101 kPa, 760 mmHg) for every 10 m (33 ft) below the surface. Even 1 m below the surface breathing through a snorkel becomes difficult because the pressure on the chest opposes inspiration. In **SCUBA diving** greater depths are made possible by pressurizing the inspired, and hence alveolar gas, to ambient pressure, but this brings other problems. Using compressed air, the increased alveolar P_{N_2} raises arterial P_{N_2}, which has effects on the brain similar to alcohol intoxication and eventually leads to **nitrogen narcosis**. Dissolved nitrogen may also cause problems if the diver surfaces too rapidly. **Decompression sickness** or **the bends** occurs when the rapidly decreased pressure causes nitrogen to come out of solution, forming bubbles in the blood and tissues, leading to musculoskeletal pains and neurological symptoms. The high pressure compresses the gas in the lungs and this expands during ascent. If the diver fails to exhale while ascending, this can rupture the lungs.

Development of the respiratory system and birth

Figure 17a Branching morphogenesis

Mesoderm

Epithelium

Signalling factors

Factors released by mesoderm cells cause the epithelium to grow inwards towards them as a bud; inhibitory factors prevent budding either side

Figure 17b Stages of lung development

Week 4 → Week 5 → Week 6 → Week 8

4th pharyngeal pouch

Laryngo-tracheal tube

Bronchial buds   Embryonic oesophagus

Trachea

Secondary bronchi

Mesoderm

Endoderm/epithelium

Segmental bronchi

Figure 17c Fetal circulation

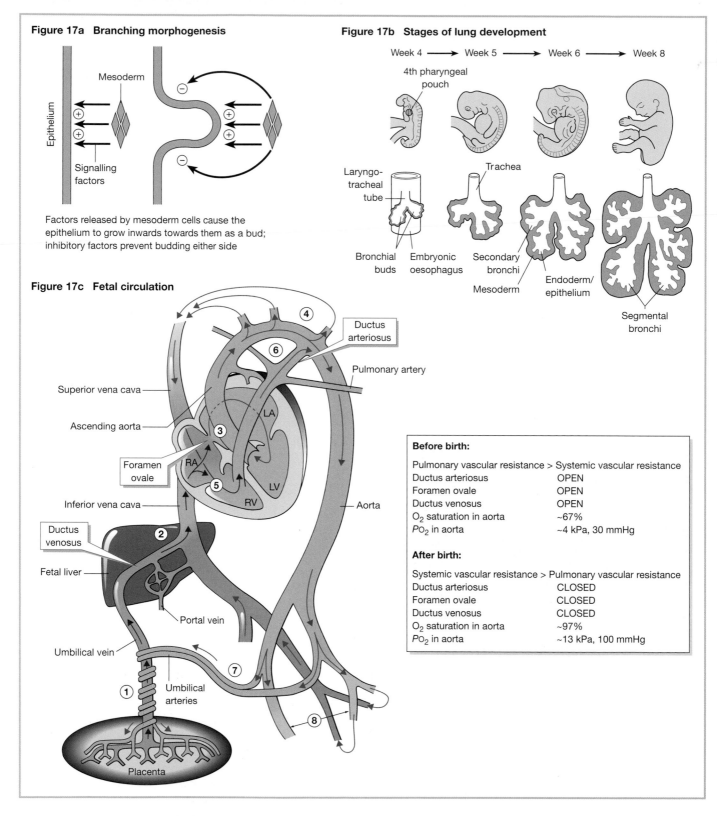

Ductus arteriosus

Pulmonary artery

Superior vena cava

Ascending aorta

LA

Foramen ovale

RA

Inferior vena cava

LV

RV

Aorta

Ductus venosus

Fetal liver

Portal vein

Umbilical vein

Umbilical arteries

Placenta

Before birth:

Pulmonary vascular resistance > Systemic vascular resistance
Ductus arteriosus   OPEN
Foramen ovale   OPEN
Ductus venosus   OPEN
O_2 saturation in aorta   ~67%
P_{O_2} in aorta   ~4 kPa, 30 mmHg

After birth:

Systemic vascular resistance > Pulmonary vascular resistance
Ductus arteriosus   CLOSED
Foramen ovale   CLOSED
Ductus venosus   CLOSED
O_2 saturation in aorta   ~97%
P_{O_2} in aorta   ~13 kPa, 100 mmHg

The Respiratory System at a Glance, Fourth Edition. Jeremy P.T. Ward. © Jeremy P.T. Ward. Published 2015 by John Wiley & Sons, Ltd.

The **embryological origins** of the lung are primitive **endoderm** of the foregut, which eventually forms the epithelium and glands of the larynx, trachea and lungs, and **splanchnic mesoderm**, which forms cartilage, smooth muscle, lung parenchyma and connective tissue. In common with many glandular organs, the lung develops by **branching morphogenesis** (Fig. 17a), with budding and branching of the endoderm/epithelium into mesoderm. The process requires reciprocal signalling between epithelium and mesoderm, with the mesoderm being primarily responsible for programming development of adjacent epithelium into the relevant structures. Many signalling molecules are vital for the orchestration of branching morphogenesis during lung development, including growth factors such as fibroblast growth factor (FGF), epidermal growth factor (EGF) and platelet-derived growth factor (PDGF); vascular endothelial growth factor (VEGF) is critical for pulmonary vascular development. Development of the respiratory system is generally divided into five stages or periods.

1 Embryonic period: The tracheobronchial tree originates from the **laryngotracheal tube**, below the fourth pharyngeal pouch at the caudal (tail) end of the primordial pharynx. The laryngotracheal tube starts to appear just prior to the fourth week of development, after the heart begins to beat. By the end of the fourth week, its end has bifurcated into two **bronchial buds**, progenitors of the two main bronchi and bronchial tree (Fig. 17b).

2 Pseudoglandular period (5–17th weeks): The bronchial buds have now developed into the primordial left and (slightly larger) right primary bronchi, which subsequently divide by branching morphogenesis into five secondary bronchi (three right, two left). At the seventh week, these have started to branch progressively into 10 (right) or 8–9 (left) **segmental** (tertiary) bronchi, each of which eventually forms a **bronchopulmonary segment**. By the 17th week, most major structures of the lung have formed and are lined with columnar epithelial cells. Conducting blood vessels are present, but the gas exchange surfaces have not yet developed and fetuses delivered during this period are therefore not viable.

3 Canalicular period (16–25th weeks): Bronchial cartilage, smooth muscle, pulmonary capillaries and connective tissue develop from the mesoderm. There is progressive differentiation and thinning of epithelial cells. The bronchi will have subdivided approximately 17 times after 24 weeks, finally forming the respiratory bronchioles which themselves divide into three to six alveolar ducts and some thin-walled **terminal sacs**. These are lined by very thin **type I alveolar pneumocytes** (squamous epithelium), which together with endothelial cells from capillaries form the future **alveolocapillary membrane** (gas exchange surface). There are a few **type II alveolar pneumocytes**, secretory epithelial cells that produce surfactant. This reduces surface tension and allows expansion of the terminal sacs/alveoli (Chapter 6), but although it is present in small amounts from about the 20th week, it is insufficient to support unaided breathing until after 26 weeks (see **neonatal respiratory distress syndrome**, Chapter 18). Some gas exchange can occur at the end of this period, as there are both thin-walled terminal sacs and good vascularization, but the general level of immaturity means that fetuses born before the end of the 24th week normally die despite intensive care.

4 Saccular (terminal sac) period (24th week to parturition): Associated with rapid development in the number of terminal sacs and the pulmonary and lymphatic capillary networks. Budding from terminal sacs and walls of terminal bronchioles and thinning of type I pneumocytes lead to formation of immature alveoli from around week 32. Sufficient surfactant and vascularization are normally present between the 24th and 26th week to allow survival of some premature fetuses, although this is very variable (Chapter 18). Surfactant increases significantly in the 2 weeks before birth.

5 Alveolar period (late fetal to childhood): Clusters of immature alveoli form during the early part of this period; mature-type alveoli with thin interalveolar septa and gas exchange surfaces do not appear until after birth. **Fetal breathing** movements are present before birth, with aspiration of amniotic fluid, and these stimulate lung growth and respiratory muscle conditioning. Lung development is impaired in the absence of fetal breathing, inadequate amniotic fluid (**oligohydramnios**) or space for lung growth (Chapter 18). The increase in lung size over the first 3 years is due primarily to an increase in number of alveoli and respiratory bronchioles; thereafter, both the number and size of alveoli increase. More than 90% of alveoli are formed after birth, reaching a maximum after 7–8 years. At the end of lung development, there are approximately 23 generations of airways, with approximately 17 million branches.

Fetal circulation and birth

Gas exchange in the fetus occurs in the **placenta**. Oxygen-rich blood from the umbilical vein flows into the liver and **ductus venosus**, and thus into the vena cava. Most blood entering the right atrium is diverted into the left atrium via the **foramen ovale**; the remainder enters the right ventricle and is pumped into the pulmonary artery as in the adult (Fig. 17c). However, the vascular resistance of the pulmonary circulation is high due to the collapsed state of the lungs and vasoconstriction, and 90% of the blood is therefore shunted via the **ductus arteriosus** into the aorta (Fig. 17c). Note that the P_aO_2 in the fetus is much lower (~4 kPa, 30 mmHg) than in the adult; oxygen transport is sustained by high-affinity fetal haemoglobin (Chapter 8).

At birth, the lungs are initially 50% full of fluid which is replaced by air. During and immediately following birth, fluid is removed via the pulmonary and lymphatic circulations, and through the mouth as a result of squeezing during delivery. Expansion and filling of the alveoli with air is critically dependent on the presence of **surfactant** to lower surface tension. The initiation of gas exchange in the lungs and consequent rise in blood P_O_2 cause vasodilatation of the pulmonary circulation and constriction of the ductus arteriosus, so that blood from the right side of the heart now follows its adult course via the lungs. The consequent fall in right atrial pressure causes the pressure gradient across the foramen ovale to reverse, causing functional closure within hours. The removal of venous return from the placenta also causes closure of the ductus venosus. Initially, pressure gradients keep the three fetal shunts closed, but after several months structural changes cause permanent closure. In 20% of adults this may remain incomplete for the foramen ovale, but is generally of no consequence.

18 Complications of development and congenital disease

Figure 18a Relationship between prematurity and development of NRDS

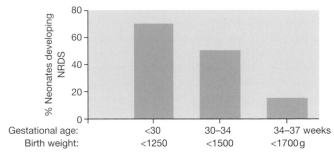

% Neonates developing NRDS

Gestational age: <30   30–34   34–37 weeks
Birth weight: <1250   <1500   <1700g

Other factors such as socioeconomic status, maternal health, race and sex also affect incidence of NRDS

Figure 18b Congenital diaphragmatic hernia

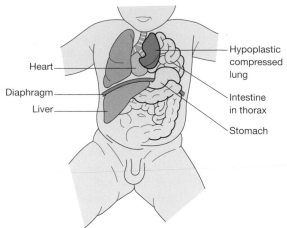

Heart

Diaphragm

Liver

Hypoplastic compressed lung

Intestine in thorax

Stomach

Figure 18c Tracheoesophageal fistula

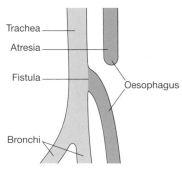

Trachea

Atresia

Fistula

Oesophagus

Bronchi

Oesophageal atresia and tracheo-oesophageal fistula (85%)

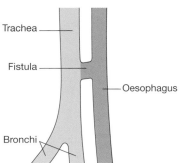

Trachea

Fistula

Oesophagus

Bronchi

Tracheo-oesophageal fistula (5%)

Figure 18d Some genetic diseases in which the lung is a primary site of injury

Disease	Inheritance	Pathogenesis	Lung pathology
Alpha$_1$-antitrypsin deficiency	AD	Protease–antiprotease imbalance	Emphysema
Ciliary dyskinesia	AR	Impaired mucociliary clearance	Airway infection, bronchiectasis
Cystic fibrosis	AR	Abnormal chloride transport	Airway infection, bronchiectasis
Familial idiopathic fibrosis	AR	Unknown	Diffuse fibrosis
Lipoid proteinosis (Urbach–Wiethe syndrome)	AR	Lipoglycoprotein deposition in upper respiratory tract causing mucosal thickening and airway obstruction	Hyalinized or granular deposits in the tracheo-bronchial submucosa
Tracheobroncho-megaly (Mounier–Kuhn syndrome)	AR	Saccular bulges between cartilage rings resulting from atrophy of elastic and smooth muscle tissue and causing impaired mucociliary clearance	Recurrent airway infections
Congenital cartilage deficiency (Williams–Campbell syndrome)	?	Deficiency of subsegmental bronchial cartilage with airway collapse	Recurrent airway infections, bronchiectasis

AD = Autosomal dominant, AR = Autosomal recessive

The Respiratory System at a Glance, Fourth Edition. Jeremy P.T. Ward. © Jeremy P.T. Ward. Published 2015 by John Wiley & Sons, Ltd.

Problems associated with premature birth

Neonatal respiratory distress syndrome (NRDS), otherwise known as hyaline membrane disease, occurs in approximately 2% of all births and is characterized by rapid, laboured breathing and often sternal retraction due to partial collapse of the lungs after each breath. Lung compliance is low. NRDS is most commonly caused by lack of sufficient quantities of surfactant and consequent high surface tension in the alveoli and small airways. Incidence therefore increases sharply with the degree of prematurity (Fig. 18a), although other factors may also reduce production of surfactant. When a premature birth is anticipated, the expectant mother can be treated with **corticosteroids** (betamethasone) to speed up fetal lung development and surfactant production. Treatment with **exogenous surfactant** in the first 30 minutes after birth, either of natural origin or artificial, has also proved to be beneficial. Survival of neonates with NRDS often requires high positive-pressure mechanical ventilation and high levels of oxygen.

The large majority of NRDS cases are related to prematurity, with some due to other causes including damage to type II pneumocytes. A very few cases are due to a congenital absence of **pulmonary surfactant protein B**. These patients do not respond to any form of therapy and tend to die in the first few months of life.

Bronchopulmonary dysplasia (chronic lung disease of the newborn) is a long-term consequence of NRDS, primarily as a result of treatment with high positive-pressure ventilation combined with high levels of oxygen (hyperoxia). The condition is characterized by alterations in the structure and function of airways and pulmonary blood vessels, including increases in airway and vascular smooth muscle and obliteration of some microstructures. This leads to poorly reversible airway obstruction and sometimes pulmonary hypertension (high pulmonary blood pressure). Survivors may retain symptoms for many years, if not for life. There are several similarities to chronic obstructive pulmonary disease (COPD; Chapter 28) and chronic severe asthma in adults.

Several techniques have been designed to minimize the incidence of bronchopulmonary dysplasia in infants with NRDS. These include extracorporeal membrane oxygenation (**ECMO**), where blood is circulated via external apparatus for gas exchange; mechanical ventilation and hyperoxia are therefore not required and some success has been reported. ECMO has also been found useful in some adults with acute respiratory distress syndrome (ARDS; Chapter 43). **Partial fluid ventilation**, where the lungs are ventilated with fluids containing oxygen-carrying perfluorocarbons, has also been reported to be beneficial. Fluid ventilation circumvents problems associated with high surface tension by removing the air–liquid interface and allows small airways to open and contribute to gas exchange.

Congenital diseases

Congenital diaphragmatic hernia is the most common cause of lung hypoplasia (inadequate development of the lung), with an incidence of about one in 2000 births. Failure of the diaphragm to fuse with the membranes on the thoracic and peritoneal wall leads to a posterolateral defect, most commonly occurring on the left side (~85%), through which the abdominal viscera pass (herniate) into the thorax (Fig. 18b). This often includes the stomach, spleen and much of the intestines. The presence of the resultant mass severely restricts lung development and later inflation, leading to a significantly reduced lung volume and life-threatening breathing difficulties. The latter are the prime cause of death in congenital diaphragmatic hernia, and most infants will die because the lungs are insufficiently developed to support life outside the uterus. Although surgical correction of the defect is possible both before and after birth, the mortality rate is very high. A related but very much less common condition is **eventration of the diaphragm**, where half the diaphragm lacks adequate muscle and bulges (eventrates) into the thoracic cavity. The viscera are forced into the pocket so formed, again restricting lung development.

Tracheoesophageal fistula (an opening between oesophagus and trachea) is the most common abnormality of the lower respiratory tract itself, with an incidence of about one in 4000 births. Its origins are located in the fourth week of development, when the embryonic respiratory tract starts to develop and divide from the embryonic oesophagus (Chapter 17). Eighty-five per cent of cases are associated with the descending part of the oesophagus having a blind ending (**oesophageal atresia**) (Fig. 18c); the lower part of the oesophagus joins instead to the base of the trachea. As a result, normal feeding is impossible and the gut becomes distended with air. There are also consequences in utero, as normally amniotic fluid is ingested by the fetus. Thus, oesophageal atresia is commonly associated with excess amniotic fluid (**polyhydramnios**), which can lead to severe defects in the central nervous system. Some 5% of cases of tracheoesophageal fistula show no atresia but only a fistula, and the remainder less common variations. Rare defects involving blockage or narrowing of the trachea itself (**tracheal atresia/ stenosis**) are nearly always accompanied by various types of tracheoesophageal fistula.

There are many **inherited disorders of haemoglobin synthesis**. In some (e.g. **thalassaemia**) there is inadequate production of the normal globin chains, and in others (e.g. HbS in **sickle cell disease**) there is production of globin chains with an abnormal amino acid sequence. They produce a variety of clinical problems mostly related to anaemia and/or alteration in the solubility (HbS) or oxygen affinity of the abnormal haemoglobin (Chapter 8).

Congenital influences on respiratory disease: several important respiratory diseases that are discussed in detail in other chapters have definite or implied genetic components, including asthma (Chapter 26), COPD (Chapter 28), emphysema (Chapter 28), cystic fibrosis (Chapter 36) and pulmonary arterial hypertension (Chapter 29). Other genetically linked diseases that cause pathological problems primarily in the lung are listed in Figure 18d.

19 Lung defence mechanisms

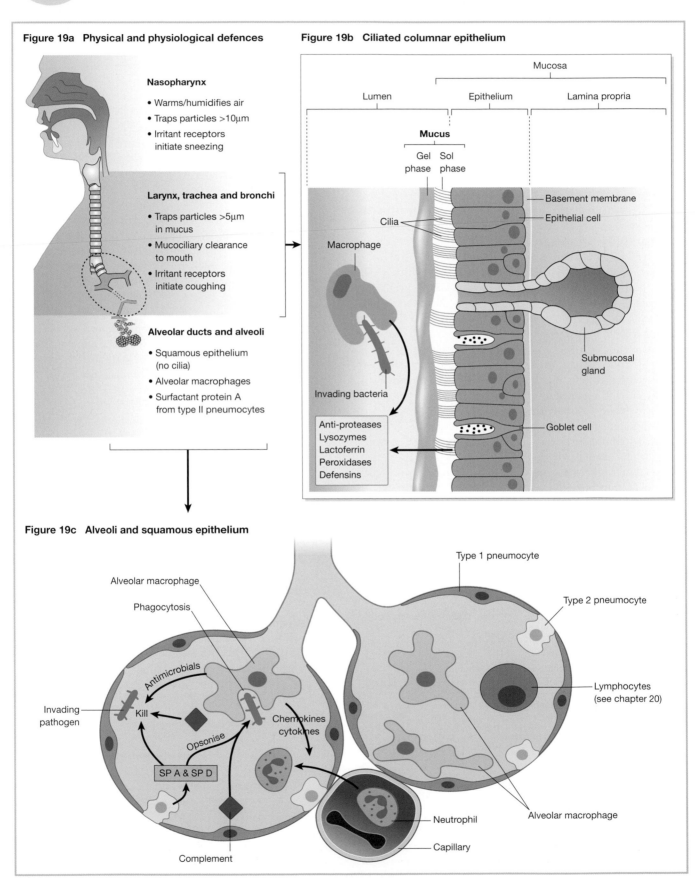

Figure 19a Physical and physiological defences

Nasopharynx

- Warms/humidifies air
- Traps particles >10µm
- Irritant receptors initiate sneezing

Larynx, trachea and bronchi

- Traps particles >5µm in mucus
- Mucociliary clearance to mouth
- Irritant receptors initiate coughing

Alveolar ducts and alveoli

- Squamous epithelium (no cilia)
- Alveolar macrophages
- Surfactant protein A from type II pneumocytes

Figure 19b Ciliated columnar epithelium

Mucosa

Lumen | Epithelium | Lamina propria

Mucus

Gel phase | Sol phase

Basement membrane
Epithelial cell
Cilia
Macrophage
Invading bacteria
Submucosal gland
Anti-proteases
Lysozymes
Lactoferrin
Peroxidases
Defensins
Goblet cell

Figure 19c Alveoli and squamous epithelium

Type 1 pneumocyte
Type 2 pneumocyte
Alveolar macrophage
Phagocytosis
Antimicrobials
Invading pathogen
Kill
Opsonise
Chemokines cytokines
SP A & SP D
Complement
Lymphocytes (see chapter 20)
Alveolar macrophage
Neutrophil
Capillary

The Respiratory System at a Glance, Fourth Edition. Jeremy P.T. Ward. © Jeremy P.T. Ward. Published 2015 by John Wiley & Sons, Ltd.

Inhalation allows ingress of dust, irritant particles and pathogens. The huge surface area of the airways provides multiple opportunities for infections and damage, and the warm humid environment provides ideal conditions for bacterial, fungal and other infestations. The respiratory tract has a range of powerful defence mechanisms, dysfunction of which underlie or contribute to many respiratory diseases. This chapter deals with *non-specific* defence mechanisms; Chapter 20 deals with the adaptive immune response.

Physical and physiological defences

The nasopharynx provides a physical barrier to particles greater than 10 μm, in the form of hairs and mucus to which particles adhere (Fig. 19a). Only particles less than 5 μm generally get further than the trachea. **Mucociliary transport** (see below) transfers particles stuck to mucus to the pharynx, where they are ingested. The nasopharynx also provides **humidifying** and **warming** functions for inhaled air, preventing drying of epithelium. Irritant particles in the nose and trachea, whether inhaled or transported from distal regions by mucociliary transport, stimulate irritant receptors (Chapter 13), provoking sneezing and coughing to eject foreign matter.

The airways are lined by epithelial cells which provide a physical barrier and secrete mucus, antimicrobial compounds, **cytokines** (signalling molecules) and **chemokines** (chemoattractants) which recruit inflammatory cells (**chemotaxis**). They can also act as **antigen-presenting cells** (Chapter 20). The epithelium of conducting airways consists of a pseudostratified layer of ciliated columnar cells interspersed with goblet and secretory (Clara) cells (Fig. 19b). Alveoli are lined with very thin, unciliated squamous epithelial cells (**type 1 pneumocytes**) to facilitate gas exchange; cuboidal **type 2 pneumocytes** secrete **surfactant** (Fig. 19c, Chapter 6).

Airway fluids and mucus

The respiratory epithelium is covered with a 5–10 μm layer of periciliary fluid (**sol phase**), which is in turn covered by a 2–15 μm layer of gelatinous mucus (**gel phase**) (Fig. 19b). Mucus is produced by **goblet cells** in the epithelium and **submucosal glands** (Fig. 19b). Its major constituents are carbohydrate-rich glycoproteins called mucins which give mucus its gel-like nature. The fluidity and ionic composition of the sol phase are regulated by epithelial ion channels and transporters, including the **cystic fibrosis transmembrane conductance regulator** (CFTR). **Cilia** on epithelial cells beat synchronously, and as they do their tips catch in the gel phase, causing it to move towards the mouth, transporting embedded particles (**mucociliary transport** or clearance). It takes ~40 minutes for mucus from large bronchi to reach the pharynx but days from the respiratory bronchioles.

Many factors disrupt mucociliary transport, including increased mucus viscosity or thickness, making it harder to move (e.g. inflammation, asthma), changes in the sol phase that inhibit cilia movement or prevent attachment to the gel phase, and defects in cilia activity (**cilia dyskinesia**). Mucociliary transport is impaired by smoking, pollutants, anaesthetics and infection. In **cystic fibrosis** dysfunction of CFTR leads to dehydration of the sol phase and mucus, increasing viscosity (Chapter 36). The rare congenital immotile cilia syndrome is due to a defective cilia 'motor' protein. Reduced mucociliary transport promotes recurrent respiratory infections that progressively damage the lungs, causing for example **bronchiectasis**, where the bronchial walls are thickened, dilated and inflamed (Chapter 36 and Case 5).

Mucus contains factors produced by epithelial and other cells or that are derived from plasma. **Antiproteases** such as α_1-**antitrypsin** inhibit the action of proteases, trypsin and elastase released from bacteria and neutrophils which degrade proteins and could damage the airways; α_1-**antitrypsin deficiency** predisposes to disruption of elastin and development of emphysema (Chapter 28). **Lysozyme** from granulocytes and epithelial cells has antifungal and bactericidal properties; together with the antimicrobial proteins lactoferrin, peroxidases and β-defensins it provides a non-specific first line of defence. The **surfactant proteins** SP A and D enhance phagocytosis by macrophages and neutrophils by coating or **opsonizing** (literally 'making ready to eat') bacteria and invasive particles, and have direct antimicrobial activity.

The airways also contain **complement**, a non-cellular defence mechanism comprised of a cascade of several proteins. These derive from the liver and enter the airways from the blood, especially in inflammation, though some can be made by macrophages and monocytes. Activated complement opsonizes pathogens thus facilitating phagocytosis, and recruits phagocytes to dispose of them; it also kills bacteria by membrane rupture. Complement is activated by surface markers (e.g. bacterial mannose) or antibodies that have 'tagged' a pathogen or material as foreign (Chapter 20).

Phagocytes and natural killers

Macrophages ('big eaters') are mobile **mononuclear phagocytes** formed by differentiation of monocytes. They act as sentinels within the airways, providing innate protection against inhaled microbes and invasive particles by **phagocytosis** and production of antimicrobial agents including lyozymes, defensins and oxygen radicals. Phagocytosed organic material is usually digested, whereas inorganic material is sequestered inside the cell. As alveolar epithelium has no cilia, alveolar macrophages are essential for removing material and cell debris, and are the major cell present within the alveoli (Fig. 19c). Macrophages also act as antigen-presenting cells (Chapter 20), but normally suppress unnecessary immune responses by producing **anti-inflammatory cytokines** such as interleukin-10 (IL-10). However, in heavy infections macrophages and epithelial cells release proinflammatory cytokines (e.g. IL-1, TNFα) and chemokines (e.g. leukotriene B$_4$, IL-8), promoting massive infiltration of **neutrophils**. Neutrophils are highly mobile leukocytes of the polymorphonuclear family (**PMNs**) which includes eosinophils and basophils, and play a key role in the innate response to bacterial infection. Neutrophils eliminate microbes by phagocytosis and release of oxygen radicals and cytotoxic proteins, including proteinases, lyozymes and defensins. Sustained activity can thus damage host tissue. Unlike macrophages, neutrophils do not ingest cell debris or inorganic material.

Activation of phagocytes by pathogens is mediated by **phagocyte pattern recognition receptors** (PRRs) including Toll-like (TLR) and C-type lectin (CLR) receptors. These recognize **pathogen-associated molecular patterns** (PAMPs) including bacterial mannose residues, viral RNA and fungal glucans. Other phagocyte receptors recognize complement-opsonized immune complexes and antigen-bound immunoglobulins (Fc receptors). Injured, infected or cancerous cells express PAMP-like molecules recognized by **natural killer** (NK) lymphocytes, which kill the cells and recruit macrophages to remove the debris.

20 Immunology of the lung

Figure 20a   Activation, differentiation and function of T cells

Polarisation of T cells into sub-types depends on antigen type and cytokines from antigen presenting cells, T_H cells, and other immune cells including macrophages, mast cells, NK cells, neutrophils, basophils and eosinophils.

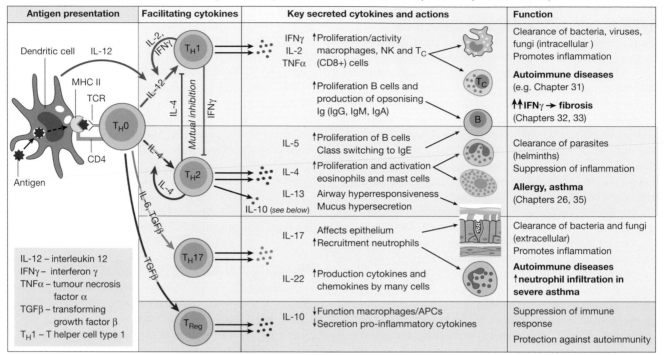

Antigen presentation	Facilitating cytokines	Key secreted cytokines and actions	Function
Dendritic cell IL-12 MHC II TCR T_H0 CD4 Antigen	IL-2, IFNγ T_H1 IL-12 IL-4 Mutual inhibition IFNγ	IFNγ IL-2 TNFα ↑Proliferation/activity macrophages, NK and T_C (CD8+) cells ↑Proliferation B cells and production of opsonising Ig (IgG, IgM, IgA)	Clearance of bacteria, viruses, fungi (intracellular) Promotes inflammation **Autoimmune diseases** (e.g. Chapter 31) ↑↑IFNγ → fibrosis (Chapters 32, 33)
IL-12 – interleukin 12 IFNγ – interferon γ TNFα – tumour necrosis factor α TGFβ – transforming growth factor β T_H1 – T helper cell type 1	IL-4 IL-4 T_H2 IL-4 IL-6, TGFβ TGFβ	IL-5 ↑Proliferation of B cells Class switching to IgE IL-4 ↑Proliferation and activation eosinophils and mast cells IL-13 Airway hyperresponsiveness IL-10 (see below) Mucus hypersecretion	Clearance of parasites (helminths) Suppression of inflammation **Allergy, asthma** (Chapters 26, 35)
	T_H17	IL-17 Affects epithelium ↑Recruitment neutrophils IL-22 ↑Production cytokines and chemokines by many cells	Clearance of bacteria and fungi (extracellular) Promotes inflammation **Autoimmune diseases** **↑neutrophil infiltration in severe asthma**
	T_{Reg}	IL-10 ↓Function macrophages/APCs ↓Secretion pro-inflammatory cytokines	Suppression of immune response Protection against autoimmunity

Figure 20b   Antibodies

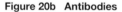

Antigen binding sites
Hypervariable regions
F_{ab}
Light chain
F_c
Heavy chain

F_c differs between classes, and binds to class-specific F_c receptors on immune cells, and also complement

Classes: mostly monomers
IgG Most common (80%)
IgE Anti-helminth, binds to and primes mast cells in allergy
IgA Mucosal immunity in airways and gut, dimer
IgM Naïve B cell antigen receptor; Secreted as a pentamer, a strong activator of complement, in T cell independent humoral responses
(**IgD** Naïve B cell antigen receptor?)

Class switching:
Activated B cells can switch the class of antibody they make, e.g. from IgM to IgG or IgE. This is regulated by T_H cytokines. Plasma cells cannot class switch, being pre-programmed

Figure 20c   Humoral immunity

Figure 20d   Cell-mediated immunity

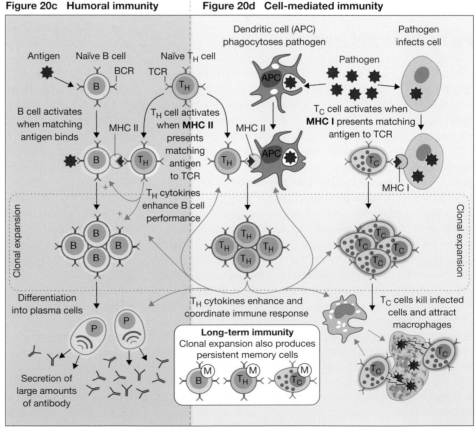

Antigen   Naïve B cell   BCR
Naïve T_H cell   TCR

B cell activates when matching antigen binds

MHC II

T_H cell activates when **MHC II** presents matching antigen to TCR

T_H cytokines enhance B cell performance

Clonal expansion

Differentiation into plasma cells

Secretion of large amounts of antibody

Dendritic cell (APC) phagocytoses pathogen
Pathogen infects cell

APC   Pathogen

MHC II

T_C cell activates when **MHC I** presents matching antigen to TCR

APC   MHC I

T_H cytokines enhance and coordinate immune response

T_C cells kill infected cells and attract macrophages

Clonal expansion

Long-term immunity
Clonal expansion also produces persistent memory cells
B(M) T_H(M) T_C(M)

The Respiratory System at a Glance, Fourth Edition. Jeremy P.T. Ward. © Jeremy P.T. Ward. Published 2015 by John Wiley & Sons, Ltd.

C hapter 19 describes non-specific defence mechanisms in the lungs. This chapter provides a basic introduction to **adaptive** immune mechanisms, which though slower are highly specific and involve **lymphocytes** and **immunoglobulins** (*antibodies*).

Immunoglobulin basics

Immunoglobulins are at the heart of adaptive immunity. Synthesized by **lymphocytes**, they recognize highly specific molecular patterns (**epitopes**) on target molecules (**antigens**). Immunoglobulins within **B cell receptors** (BCR) and **T cell receptors** (TCR) allow B and T lymphocytes (see below) to recognize their specific antigen and consequently activate. Only B and plasma cells secrete immunoglobulins (IgM, IgG, IgA, IgE) into the extracellular fluid (see **humoral immunity**). All immunoglobulin classes have a constant region (F_C) attached to two *hypervariable* branches (F_{ab}) which recognize the epitope (Fig. 20b). Random mutations in F_{ab} during lymphocyte maturation provide $>10^8$ F_{ab} variants, sufficient to match any antigen likely to be encountered. **Allelic exclusion** ensures each mature lymphocyte expresses only one immunoglobulin variant, but the large number of lymphocytes and random nature of production ensures every variant is expressed, if only in a few cells. Lymphocytes directed against *self* are (normally) destroyed during maturation. Groups of lymphocytes expressing the same F_{ab} variant are called **clones**.

Lymphocytes

Lymphocytes develop from common bone marrow progenitors. **B lymphocytes** (B cells) mature in lymphoid tissues and bone marrow, and are responsible for **humoral immunity**. **T lymphocytes** (T cells) mature in the thymus and provide **cell-mediated immunity**, but also facilitate humoral responses. BCR respond to extracellular antigens and can recognize any type of antigens (e.g. protein/peptide, polysaccharide, lipids). TCR only recognize peptides, which must be presented by B cells or **antigen-presenting cells** (APC) via their surface **major histocompatibility complex** (**MHC II**) (Fig. 20a); MHC II displays peptides retained within vesicles following internalisation and processing (B cells), or phagocytosis (APCs). APCs include **dendritic cells**, **macrophages, B cells** and sometimes epithelial cells. Naïve (mature but not yet activated) antigen-specific lymphocytes recirculate between lymphoid tissues, though some are present in the mucosa and alveoli. Lymphocytes activate on encountering a matching antigen, and undergo **clonal expansion** – rapid proliferation resulting in a large number of identical cells with the same immunoglobulin variant. **Memory** B and T cells which persist for years are also produced during clonal expansion. These respond more rapidly and powerfully to subsequent exposures to the same antigen, and provide long-term immunity. In chronic infections bronchus-associated lymphoid tissue (**BALT**) may develop where B cells can mature and proliferate.

Helper T cells (T_H, also called CD4+ because they express CD4, a co-receptor for MHC II) play a critical coordinating role in the immune response. They assist maturation of B cells, release immunomodulatory cytokines, and activate APC and other cells. Naïve T_H cells (T_H0) differentiate on activation into sub-types according to stimulus and local cytokines; they are distinguished by function and their signature cytokines (Fig. 20a). T_H1 cells enable **cell-mediated immunity** and target intracellular bacteria and protozoa; they induce inflammation and enhance phagocytosis by macrophages and proliferation of **cytotoxic T cells** (T_C, CD8+; see below). T_H2 cells facilitate **humoral immunity** and target extracellular pathogens and parasites (helminths), but also underlie **allergy**; they induce B cell **class switching** towards **IgE** and stimulate B cells, **eosinophils** and **mast cells** (Chapter 26). Notably, T_H2 cytokines suppress T_H1 and promote T_H2 responses, and vice versa, tending to preserve the *status quo*. Inappropriate switching to T_H2 may underlie allergy. T_H17 cells target extracellular bacteria and fungi; both T_H17 and T_H1 are implicated in autoimmune and chronic inflammatory diseases (e.g. Chapters 33, 34). **Regulatory T cells** (T_{Reg}) suppress immune responses.

Adaptive response

Humoral immunity (Fig. 20c): When a naïve B cell recognizes a matching extracellular antigen it undergoes clonal expansion before differentiating into **plasma cells**. These switch from expressing BCR to secreting massive amounts of antigen-specific IgM, IgG, IgA or IgE into the extracellular fluid. For non-protein antigens the process is **T cell independent**. Protein antigens binding to BCR are internalized and processed to peptides, which are presented to T_H cells via MHC II. When antigen and TCR match, T_H cells proliferate and releases cytokines (e.g. **IL-2**) which strongly potentiate B cell proliferation and function of plasma cells.

Extracellular immunoglobulins neutralize toxins, prevent attachment of viruses, and opsonize or agglutinate (clump together) antigen-bearing pathogens for phagocytosis (Chapter 19). The antigen-immunoglobulin complex activates **complement** (Chapter 19), and **phagocytes** (e.g. macrophages, neutrophils) via their F_C receptors. IgM is first to be produced in an infection and is the main effector of T cell-independent humoral immunity; its pentameric structure provides a particularly strong activator of complement. **IgG** production starts later, but IgG is very long lasting and the most abundant immunoglobulin in health, providing sustained immunity. **Secretory IgA** dimers bind to a **secretory component** on epithelial cells, which enables transfer across epithelia; it is present in large quantities within airway fluids and blocks entry of pathogens. **IgE** is least abundant in plasma because it avidly attaches to IgE-specific F_C receptors on **mast cells** and basophils, thus priming them as sentinels. Antigen binding causes cross-linking of two IgE, initiating cell activation. Mast cells degranulate, releasing large amounts of histamine and other mediators (Chapter 26), whilst basophils release T_H2 cytokines. Though targeted at parasites (e.g. helminths), this mechanism also underlies **type 1 hypersensitivity** in allergy and asthma (Chapter 26). In allergic individuals specific IgEs may be greatly raised.

Cell-mediated immunity (Fig. 20d): After APCs (dendritic cells, macrophages) phagocytose pathogens (Chapter 19), some migrate to lymphoid tissues and present associated antigens to naïve T_H cells (via MHC II). On antigen recognition, T_H cells proliferate and release type-dependent cytokines that stimulate other immune cells (APCs, T_H, T_C, NK, mast cells, granulocytes), including B and plasma cells (thus also inducing a humoral response). T_C **cells** however detect *cytosolic* antigens presented by **MHC I** on virally infected or tumorous cells, or APCs; unlike MHC II, MHC I is present on all cells. T_C cells then proliferate and kill infected cells by inducing apoptosis.

History, examination and investigation

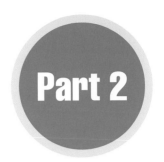

21 History and examination

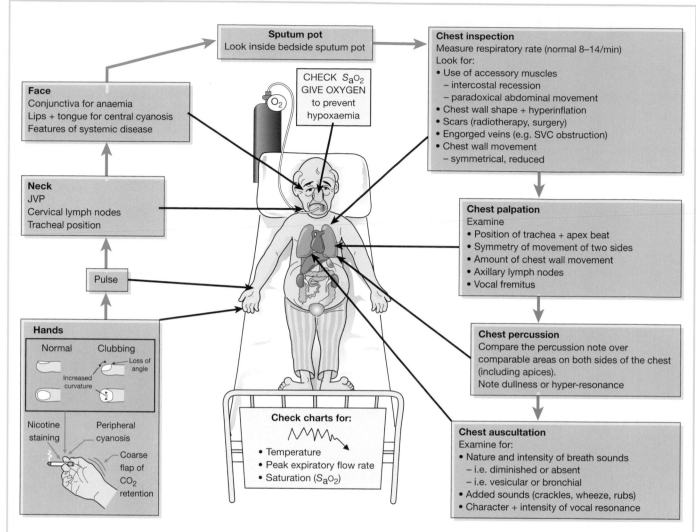

Sputum pot
Look inside bedside sputum pot

CHECK S_aO_2 GIVE OXYGEN to prevent hypoxaemia

Face
Conjunctiva for anaemia
Lips + tongue for central cyanosis
Features of systemic disease

Neck
JVP
Cervical lymph nodes
Tracheal position

Pulse

Hands

Normal   Clubbing
Loss of angle
Increased curvature

Nicotine staining   Peripheral cyanosis
Coarse flap of CO_2 retention

Check charts for:
• Temperature
• Peak expiratory flow rate
• Saturation (S_aO_2)

Chest inspection
Measure respiratory rate (normal 8–14/min)
Look for:
• Use of accessory muscles
  – intercostal recession
  – paradoxical abdominal movement
• Chest wall shape + hyperinflation
• Scars (radiotherapy, surgery)
• Engorged veins (e.g. SVC obstruction)
• Chest wall movement
  – symmetrical, reduced

Chest palpation
Examine
• Position of trachea + apex beat
• Symmetry of movement of two sides
• Amount of chest wall movement
• Axillary lymph nodes
• Vocal fremitus

Chest percussion
Compare the percussion note over comparable areas on both sides of the chest (including apices).
Note dullness or hyper-resonance

Chest auscultation
Examine for:
• Nature and intensity of breath sounds
  – i.e. diminished or absent
  – i.e. vesicular or bronchial
• Added sounds (crackles, wheeze, rubs)
• Character + intensity of vocal resonance

Table 1 Causes of clubbing

Common:
Bronchial carcinoma
Suppurative lung infection
  – bronchiectasis
  – lung abscess
  – empyema
Interstitial fibrosis

Uncommon:
Bacterial endocarditis
Cyanotic heart disease
Inflammatory bowel disease
Malabsorption
Atrial myxoma
Cirrhosis
FamilialIdiopathic
Pleural mesothelioma

Table 2 Typical physical signs associated with specific respiratory disorders

Disorder	Chest wall movement	Percussion note	Breath sounds	Added sounds
Consolidation	↓On affected side	↓ Dull	Bronchial	Coarse crackles
Collapse	↓↓On affected side	↓ Dull	Absent or bronchial	None
Pleural effusion	↓On affected side	↓↓ Stony dull	Diminished*	None (±rub)
Interstitial fibrosis	↓On both sides	Normal or ± ↓	Vesicular or diminished	Fine inspiratory crackles
Pneumothorax	↓On affected side	Normal or hyper-resonant	Diminished**	None
Asthma/COPD	↓On both sides	Normal	Vesicular with prolonged expiration	Expiratory wheeze

* Bronchial breathing may occur above the effusion; ** an audible click (in time with cardiac systole) may occur on the left side

The Respiratory System at a Glance, Fourth Edition. Jeremy P.T. Ward. © Jeremy P.T. Ward. Published 2015 by John Wiley & Sons, Ltd.

History

A comprehensive history exploring the time course, nature and severity of symptoms is the most important factor in establishing the cause of respiratory (or any other) disease. A systematic logical approach is outlined below and ensures a thorough, complete enquiry.

1 General features: age, sex, race and marital status are recorded as these may be associated with specific diseases. Thus, tuberculosis (TB) is more common in Asians, sarcoidosis in Afro-Caribbeans.

2 Presenting complaint: lists the main symptoms, usually chest pain, breathlessness, cough or haemoptysis in respiratory disease.

3 History of the presenting complaint: explores the specific features (e.g. onset and progress) of the main symptoms and associated systemic manifestations (e.g. fever, rigors, night sweats, malaise, weight loss, lymphadenopathy, arthritis and rashes). Thus, drenching night sweats and weight loss are associated with TB and cancer and erythema nodosum (inflammatory skin nodules) with sarcoidosis or TB. Obstructive sleep apnoea causes daytime sleepiness and is associated with snoring, obesity and collar size of more than 17 in. (43 cm).

- *Chest pain:* establish site, sort (pleuritic, aching), severity, onset (gradual, sudden), periodicity (intermittent, constant), duration (minutes, days), aggravating and relieving factors (i.e. worse/better with breathing, posture) and time off work. Pleuritic pain is a localized, sharp pain aggravated by deep breathing.
- *Breathlessness:* occurs at rest, on exercise or when lying flat (orthopnoea). Determine rate of onset (sudden, gradual), when it occurs (i.e. nocturnal), exercise tolerance (i.e. when walking, running or climbing stairs) and associated symptoms (e.g. hayfever, wheeze and stridor). In chronic obstructive pulmonary disease (COPD) breathlessness is worse on exercise. In contrast, breathlessness due to pulmonary oedema may suddenly wake a sleeping (i.e. supine) patient with heart failure. Nocturnal breathlessness with wheeze or seasonal breathlessness with hayfever suggests asthma.
- *Cough:* in the morning indicates chronic bronchitis (smoker's cough), at night suggests asthma or may be persistent after viral respiratory tract infections with bronchial hyperresponsiveness. Cough may be dry or productive of sputum. In a smoker, persistent cough, change in character or a bovine cough (due to recurrent laryngeal nerve palsy) indicates development of bronchial carcinoma.
- *Sputum:* morning cough and sputum production for 3 months a year for more than 1 year defines chronic bronchitis. Yellow or green, mucopurulent sputum occurs in chest infections and when copious and foul smelling may indicate bronchiectasis. Pink frothy sputum is typical of pulmonary oedema.
- *Haemoptysis:* determine frequency and quantity (i.e. flecks in sputum, fresh red blood); more than 500 mL haemoptysis in 24 hours is life-threatening. Infection (e.g. TB, pneumonia, bronchiectasis and *Aspergillus)* accounts for approximately 80% of haemoptysis; bronchial carcinoma and rarer causes (e.g. pulmonary infarction, vasculitis) for approximately 20%.

4 Past medical history: enquire about previous respiratory conditions; childhood whooping cough is associated with adult bronchiectasis; TB may reactivate in later life. Atopy and eczema are often associated with asthma. Assess understanding of current diseases and compliance with medications. Review previous chest X-rays, hospital admissions and the need for mechanical ventilation.

5 Medications: review current and previous medications, including inhalers, nebulizers and oxygen. Determine whether recent changes are associated with new symptoms (e.g. β-blockers may precipitate or worsen asthma; cytotoxics (e.g. methotrexate) can cause pulmonary fibrosis). Record allergies to medications and foods.

6 Family, occupational and social history: a family history of atopy, TB, COPD or cystic fibrosis may help establish a diagnosis. **Smoking history** including duration and amount (1 pack/day for 1 year = 1 pack/year). **Alcohol abuse** predisposes to TB. **Occupation** may predispose to respiratory disease (e.g. asbestos exposure is associated with pleural plaques, fibrosis and mesothelioma; isocyanate exposure with asthma). **Environmental** factors may be important (e.g. pet birds may cause psittacosis). **Travel** is associated with specific infections (e.g. Legionnaire's disease).

Examination

Detection of typical constellations of clinical signs helps establish a diagnosis, although poor interobserver agreement questions their reliability and emphasizes the need for other investigations (Fig. 21).

General examination

Determine if the patient is well or unwell and whether breathing, airway and circulation are adequate. Examine breathing rate and pattern. Assess the degree of breathlessness at rest or while undressing. Check observation charts (e.g. temperature and S_aO_2) and bedside sputum pots. Note general features such as obesity, cachexia, jaundice, respiratory distress, anxiety and pain. Examine

- *Hands:* for nicotine staining, finger clubbing (Fig. 21: Table 1), peripheral cyanosis, the fine tremor of excessive β_2-agonist therapy and the coarse tremor of a CO_2 retention flap. A 'bounding' pulse also suggests CO_2 retention.
- *Face and neck:* for lymph nodes and features of systemic diseases. Examine the conjunctiva for anaemia and the tongue (lips) for central cyanosis (blue discoloration due to an increase in deoxygenated arterial haemoglobin). Measure the jugular venous pressure (JVP) and changes with respiration (i.e. fixed and raised in superior vena cava (SVC) obstruction). Check for tracheal deviation and stridor (inspiratory wheeze due to upper airway obstruction).

Chest examination

Includes anterior and posterior inspection, palpation, percussion and auscultation, with comparison of the left and right sides. The pattern of physical signs will indicate likely diagnoses (Table 2).

- *Inspection:* includes chest and spinal shape, scars of previous radiotherapy or surgery, subcutaneous nodules, engorged chest wall veins (SVC obstruction), hyperinflation, symmetry of chest wall movement and use of accessory muscles of respiration.
- *Palpation:* examine for tenderness, apex beat position and adequate chest wall expansion (>3 cm).
- *Percussion:* assess for dullness and hyper-resonance.
- *Auscultation:* assess breath sounds and their distribution including nature (i.e. vesicular, bronchial), intensity (i.e. absent, diminished) and added sounds (wheezes, crackles, rub). **'Vesicular' breath sounds** are normal inspiratory and expiratory sounds; there is no gap between inspiration and expiration. **Bronchial breath sounds** are high-pitched ('blowing') sounds with a gap between inspiration and expiration. They occur with consolidation, collapse and above pleural effusions. Reduced breath sounds occur with effusions, consolidation, pneumothorax and raised diaphragm. **Crepitations** may be fine, fixed and inspiratory due to pulmonary fibrosis or early consolidation, or coarse due to excessive bronchial secretions (e.g. bronchiectasis). **Vocal resonance** and **tactile vocal fremitus** increase over areas of consolidation and diminish over effusions and collapsed lung.

46

Part 2 History, examination and investigation

22 Pulmonary function tests

Figure 22a Volume–time spirograms during forced expiration from total lung capacity

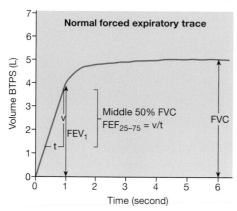

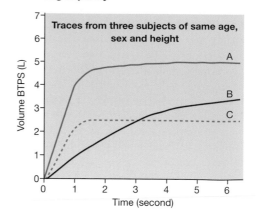

FEV$_1$ = Forced expiratory volume in 1 second

FVC = Forced vital capacity

FEF$_{25-75}$ = Mean forced expiratory flow from
25–75% of FVC

A = Normal respiratory system

B = Obstructive airway disease

C = Restrictive lung disease

Figure 22b Helium dilution for measuring functional residual capacity*

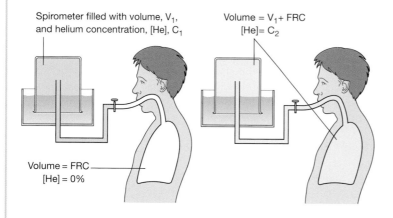

Spirometer filled with volume, V$_1$, and helium concentration, [He], C$_1$

Volume = V$_1$+ FRC
[He]= C$_2$

Volume = FRC
[He] = 0%

Starting at the end of a normal expiration (lung volume = FRC), the subject breathes in and out from the spirometer until equilibrium is reached. Since helium is poorly soluble in blood, the quantity of helium in the final spirometer – lung mixture equals that originally in the spirometer.

$$V_1 \times C_1 = (V_1 + FRC) \times C_2 \quad \therefore FRC = V_1 \times \left(\frac{C_1 - C_2}{C_2} \right)$$

*Note: To measure TLC or RV, the subject is asked to breathe in fully or breathe out fully before breathing the helium gas mixture.

Figure 22c The body plethysmograph for measuring lung volumes

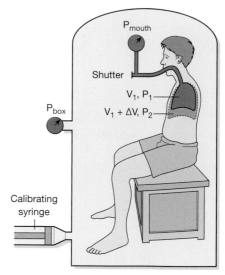

P$_{mouth}$

Shutter

V$_1$, P$_1$

V$_1$ + ΔV, P$_2$

P$_{box}$

Calibrating syringe

The subject inhales against a closed shutter

Lung volume expands from V$_1$ to V$_1$ + ΔV

ΔV can be deduced from the rise in box pressure, P$_{box}$ (calibrated with known volumes)

Mouth (= alveolar) pressure falls from P$_1$ to P$_2$

From Boyle's law: $V_1 \times P_1 = P_2 \times (V_1 + \Delta V)$

Hence the original volume in the lungs, V$_1$, can be found

The Respiratory System at a Glance, Fourth Edition. Jeremy P.T. Ward. © Jeremy P.T. Ward. Published 2015 by John Wiley & Sons, Ltd.

Accurate assessment of defects in airflow, lung volume or gas exchange is essential to the diagnosis and management of many respiratory disorders. It is important to note that these tests characterize 'defects'; the clinician has to diagnose 'diseases'. The normal range of many lung function tests is very wide, and it is essential to compare the patient's measured values with those predicted for the subject's age, height and gender using standard **nomograms** constructed from large samples of healthy individuals.

Airway resistance (Chapter 7) can be measured using a **body plethysmograph** (Fig. 22c) to measure alveolar pressure. **Lung compliance** can be measured using **oesophageal pressure** to assess intrapleural pressure (Chapter 6). More commonly, abnormalities of airway resistance (in obstructive airway disease) are assessed indirectly from forced expiratory manoeuvres, and abnormalities of compliance (in restrictive lung disease) are assessed indirectly from lung volume measurements.

Forced expiratory tests

Peak expiratory flow rate (PEFR) is frequently measured, despite its inability to distinguish between different types of ventilatory defect and its dependence on patient effort (Fig. 7c). The subject breathes out as hard and fast as possible from total lung capacity (TLC) into a meter which records the maximum momentary flow rate achieved during the expiration. Inexpensive versions of the peak flowmeter are available and used for home monitoring. It is reduced in obstructive disease, respiratory muscle weakness and often in restrictive lung disease (secondary to reduced TLC). Its main value lies in monitoring diseases, especially asthma, once the diagnosis has been made.

In contrast, plots of **volume against time (spirogram)** or **airflow against volume** during a forced expiration can help to distinguish between different types of defects. The patient is asked to inhale to TLC and breathe out as hard and fast as possible to residual volume (RV). A plot of volume against time (Fig. 22a) can be produced by continuously measuring volume, either with a bellows spirometer or by integrating a flowmeter output. If a flowmeter is used, it is also possible to compute a flow–volume plot from the same forced expiration (Fig. 7c). Flow–volume plots show characteristic shapes with different defects (Fig. 7e), such as the 'scooped out' appearance seen in obstructive airway disease.

Forced vital capacity (FVC) and **forced expiratory volume in '1' second (FEV$_1$)** can be read off the volume–time plot (Fig. 22a). FEV$_1$ is extremely reproducible and correlates well with function and prognosis. It is normal for FVC and FEV$_1$ to peak in adults in the third decade and then decline by approximately 30 mL/year (Chapter 24). Forced expiratory ratio (FER = FEV$_1$/ FVC) is normally 0.75–0.90, but higher values may occur in healthy children. FER helps distinguish between obstructive and restrictive ventilatory defects. Typically, in obstructive lung diseases (e.g. COPD and acute asthma), the FER is less than 0.70. If the airway obstruction is due to asthma, FEV$_1$, FVC and FER may all increase after the inhalation of bronchodilators. In restrictive lung disease (e.g. lung fibrosis), absolute values of FEV$_1$ and FVC are reduced, but FER is normal or high.

Forced mid-expiratory flow (FEF$_{25-75}$) is the average forced expiratory flow rate over the middle 50% of the FVC. It may be especially affected by small airway disease, but the normal range is wide.

Maximal voluntary ventilation (MVV) is measured by asking the subject to breathe as hard and fast as possible into a spirometer for 15 seconds, with the ventilation expressed in L/min. It is very dependent on effort and not very reproducible, but it may correlate well with subjective dyspnoea.

Lung volumes

Typical values for lung volumes are given in Figure 3, Table 1, for an average-sized healthy young man. Lung volumes are very variable and actual values must always be interpreted in relation to the predicted values for people of the patient's age, height and gender. Some volumes can be measured using simple spirometers and some require more sophisticated techniques. **Restrictive ventilatory defects (RVDs)** are characterized by a reduction in TLC. Lung volumes such as TLC, RV and functional residual capacity (FRC) can be measured by **helium dilution** (Fig. 22b) or by **body plethysmography** (Fig. 22c). The gas dilution method is simpler for patients, but it is sensitive to gas leaks and will underestimate TLC in the presence of extensive bullous or cystic lung disease. RVDs may be caused by parenchymal lung disease (pulmonary fibrosis, scleroderma, pulmonary oedema), chest wall disease (kyphoscoliosis, massive obesity) or weak respiratory muscles (myasthenia gravis, muscular dystrophy). RV and FRC can help distinguish between these conditions, as FRC and RV are usually reduced in lung disease; whereas FRC is usually normal in muscle weakness and RV is elevated if it also affects expiratory muscles. FVC and TLC usually decline in parallel; therefore, once an RVD has been established by measurement of TLC, the progress of the disease may be followed with FVC from spirometry.

Measurement of lung compliance (Chapter 6) and **transdiaphragmatic pressure** (P_{di}) may distinguish further between RVD due to parenchymal lung disease or muscle weakness. By using two small balloon-tipped catheters, one measuring oesophageal ($P_{pleural}$) pressure and the other gastric (P_{abd}) pressure, P_{di} (= $P_{abd} - P_{pleural}$) can be measured during a maximal inspiration or sniff from FRC. Typically, in parenchymal lung disease lung compliance is low and P_{di} normal; whereas in respiratory muscle weakness lung compliance is relatively normal and P_{di} low.

Diffusing capacity, D_L (= transfer factor, T_L), is a measure of the ability of gas to diffuse from the alveolus into pulmonary capillary blood. As discussed in Chapter 5, $D_L co$ is used as a surrogate for $D_L O_2$, since (unlike $D_L O_2$) it is possible to measure it and carbon monoxide diffuses across the lung in a fashion similar to oxygen. It often helps interpretation to normalize $D_L co$ to the alveolar volume (V_A) by calculating the coefficient, **KCO** = $D_L co/V_A$. $D_L co$ is reduced by reduced alveolar surface area, thickened alveolar–capillary membrane, reduced capillary blood volume or anaemia. Reductions in the $D_L co$ can be caused by a variety of parenchymal diseases (idiopathic pulmonary fibrosis, emphysema, pneumonia) or vascular diseases (pulmonary hypertension, pulmonary oedema), such that the test is sensitive but not specific. Reductions in the $D_L co$ below 50% predicted for age, sex and height are often associated with oxygen desaturation during exercise. Severe reductions in $D_L co$ (<20% predicted) may result in resting hypoxaemia.

Arterial blood gases ($P_a O_2$, $P_a CO_2$ and pHa) and **arterial oxygen saturation** are important tests of respiratory system function and are discussed in Chapters 25 and 45.

23 Chest imaging and bronchoscopy

Evaluation of the CXR includes all the following:

① Date: ② Name:

③ AP/PA: Is it AP (anteroposterior)
   or PA (posteroanterior)?
   (Heart size cannot be measured if AP)

④ Is it well positioned? The trachea should be
   midway between clavicles

⑤ Penetration: The disc spaces should be just
   visible through the cardiac shadows
   (underpenetrated = plethoric lungs
      overpenetrated = dark lungs)

⑥ Soft tissues and breast shadows
   (mastectomy in a female)

⑦ Right diaphragm 2 cm higher than left
   (raised when paralysed, flat in asthma/COPD)

⑧ Check ribs for fractures, metastases

⑨ Right heart border = right atrium

⑩ Hilium = bronchi, arteries and veins

⑪ Superior vena cava

(a) Chest radiograph interpretation

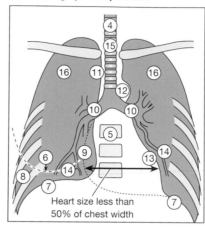

Heart size less than
50% of chest width

⑫ Aortic arch

⑬ Left heart border = left ventricle

⑭ Pulmonary vessels

⑮ Trachea and main bronchi

⑯ Lung fields

Normal chest X-ray

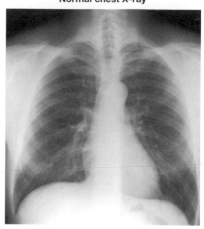

① Thoracic vertebral bodies

② Scapula

③ Pulmonary trunk and hilium

④ Descending aorta

⑤ Head of clavicle

⑥ Trachea

⑦ Arch of aorta

⑧ Ascending aorta

⑨ Anterior space (thymus)

⑩ Heart

⑪ Sternum

⑫ Diaphragm

(b) Chest radiograph interpretation

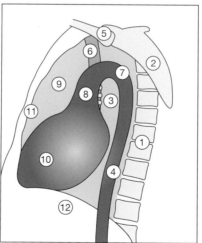

Normal lateral X-ray

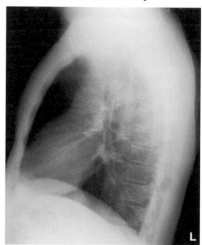

① Oesophagus

② Right lung

③ Right main bronchus

④ Right pulmonary artery and branches

⑤ Superior vena cava

⑥ Ascending aorta

⑦ Pulmonary trunk

⑧ Mediastinum and heart

⑨ Left pulmonary artery and branches

⑩ Left main bronchus

⑪ Left lung

⑫ Descending aorta

(c)

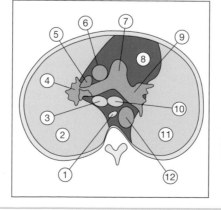

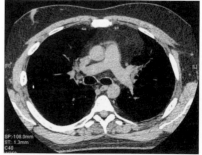

The Respiratory System at a Glance, Fourth Edition. Jeremy P.T. Ward. © Jeremy P.T. Ward. Published 2015 by John Wiley & Sons, Ltd.

Standard (two-dimensional) chest X-rays to detect, diagnose or monitor morphological abnormalities in the chest are the mainstay of thoracic radiographical imaging and account for more than 50% of procedures. Recent innovations include digital, three-dimensional computed tomography (CT) scans and physiological (positron emission tomography (PET), ventilation–perfusion scans) imaging. Specific radiographical abnormalities are discussed in individual chapters.

Posteroanterior (PA) and lateral chest radiographs (CXRs) allow two-dimensional visualization of the lungs, great vessels, heart, diaphragm and mediastinum. PA films should be performed standing in full inspiration. Routine lateral films are not required for screening purposes. Figures 23a and 23b illustrate CXR features and interpretation. Portable anterior–posterior films (AP) in patients unable to stand magnify the heart and mediastinum and do not allow detailed visualization of lung parenchyma.

A standard PA and lateral CXR should allow visualization of both lungs, including the diaphragmatic position, as well as the trachea, main carina, major bronchi, lung fissures, aorta, main pulmonary arteries and heart. Understanding of normal CXR anatomy is essential to allow recognition of abnormal lung parenchymal infiltrates, enlarged lymph nodes adjacent to the trachea or in the hila, enlarged pulmonary arteries, volume loss of a lobe or segment or cardiac enlargement. In the case of a suspected pleural effusion, lateral decubitus films allow visualization of as little as 50 mL of free-flowing fluid. Digital CXRs are being developed that allow more detailed views of the denser portions of the thorax and show finer detail of the lung parenchyma.

Computed tomography: a limitation of standard CXR imaging is that the two-dimensional image obscures details and averages densities in the third dimension (anterior–posterior on the PA film). CT allows thin slice axial images and fine-detailed examination of intrathoracic structures. It is more sensitive at detecting small lesions and in determining their relationship to other intrathoracic structures. Gross features are shown in Figure 23c. Indications for CT are:

- *Bronchial carcinoma:* to detect and assess operability and prognosis of tumours (Chapter 42) by determining location, size and the presence of abnormal lymph nodes (e.g. mediastinal and axillary).
- *Lung parenchymal disease:* to detect and localize interstitial lung infiltrates, bronchiectasis, cavities, bulla, fluid collections and airway abnormalities.
- *Mediastinal masses:* to determine extent and relationship to other structures.
- *Pleural disease:* to detect asbestos-related plaques, mesothelioma and to determine the cause of pleural effusions.
- *Pulmonary emboli (PE):* administration of intravenous contrast allows imaging of the pulmonary blood vessels and detection of emboli.

Examples of CT scans are shown in several chapters. Newer technology allows complete axial scanning of the thorax with a single breath-hold.

Ventilation–perfusion (V/Q) scans are mostly performed in the evaluation of pulmonary embolism (Chapter 30). Gamma cameras can visualize radiopharmaceuticals either injected into the venous blood (perfusion) or inhaled (ventilation). Thromboembolism classically causes a V/Q mismatch, with absence of perfusion in the presence of ventilation. Unfortunately, the value of V/Q scans is limited by the finding that many PEs result in indeterminate V/Q scans that show small mismatches or matched V/Q deficits. In these cases, other studies must be utilized to demonstrate thromboemboli. Contrast CT scans are increasingly used to detect PE (see above) and have largely superseded V/Q scanning. Quantitative V/Q scans may be used in preparation for lung resection surgery, to assess regional lung function and estimate the amount of residual lung function.

Pulmonary angiography visualizes the vasculature following injection of contrast medium (Chapter 30). It may be required in patients with suspected PE, equivocal V/Q scans, pulmonary hypertension and pulmonary vascular disease, including vasculitis and arteriovenous malformations. These studies are often preceded by echocardiography to visualize right ventricular function and estimate pulmonary artery pressure using Doppler imaging.

PET utilizes a fluorinated analogue of glucose (FDG) to give images of the lung that highlight areas of increased glucose metabolism. Malignant cells have increased glucose uptake and appear as increased densities on PET images. Recent studies have demonstrated that PET is useful in distinguishing between benign and malignant solitary pulmonary nodules and in detecting small nodal metastases that are not detected on CT scanning. For these indications, PET has a sensitivity and specificity of 80–97% with false-positive scans seen in cases of infection or granulomatous inflammation. Whole body PET has been used to detect clinically inapparent distant metastases.

Bronchoscopy enables direct visualization down to the fourth and fifth divisions of the endobronchial tree. Chest physicians perform most bronchoscopies as day cases under local anaesthetic in the sedated but awake patient, using a flexible fibre optic instrument. It has the advantages of visualization of the upper lobes and is a safe technique with a low complication rate. Saturation and heart rhythm should be monitored and supplemental oxygen should be administered during the procedure. Facilities for resuscitation should always be immediately available. Thoracic surgeons may use a rigid bronchoscope in the fully anaesthetized patient. This instrument allows larger biopsies and better suctioning, and is the method of choice when removing inhaled foreign bodies. Bronchoscopy is most frequently performed to investigate if a shadow on a CXR is due to a lung cancer (Chapter 42). If an endobronchial tumour is seen, biopsies for histological analysis and washings and brush samples for cytological analysis can be taken. In addition, information regarding the operability of the tumour can be obtained. Bronchoscopy can also be used to diagnose parenchymal lung disease using the technique of transbronchial biopsy, which obtains parenchymal and bronchial tissue for histological examination. Collection of bronchoalveolar fluid (bronchoalveolar lavage, BAL) is useful in diagnosing alveolitis (raised lymphocyte count in sarcoidosis), infection in the immunocompromised patient (e.g. *Pneumocystis jirovecii* pneumonia) and tuberculosis. Bronchoscopy also aids investigation of collapsed segments or lobes. Therapeutically, bronchoscopy is used to remove inhaled foreign bodies, to aspirate sputum plugs and secretions, to relieve stenosis by placement of stents and treat endobronchial tumours with laser or endobronchial radiotherapy. Haemorrhage, pneumothorax and cardiac arrhythmia, although uncommon, are the main complications of fibre optic bronchoscopy.

24 Public health and smoking

Figure 24a   All UK deaths in 2004

All UK deaths in 2004	587 808	
Ischaemic heart disease	106 081	
Non-respiratory cancer	122 512	
All deaths from respiratory disease	117 456	

Respiratory disease	Cases	%
• Pneumonia and TB	35 814	30.5
• Lung cancer	34 721	29.6
• Progressive non-malignant causes	35 979	30.6
– COPD + asthma	28 859	24.6
– pulmonary circulatory disease	3926	3.3
– pneumoconiosis	3024	2.6
– cystic fibrosis	139	0.1
– sarcoidosis	31	0.03
• Others (congenital etc.)	10 527	9

Figure 24c   Total UK emergency medical admissions by diagnosis (2004)

COPD	111 000
Angina	79 000
CCF	62 000
Pneumonia	57 000
Gastroenteritis	54 000
Diabetes + complications	18 000

Figure 24b   Progressive decline in lung function in smokers and non-smokers and the effect of stopping smoking at 45 and 65 years old

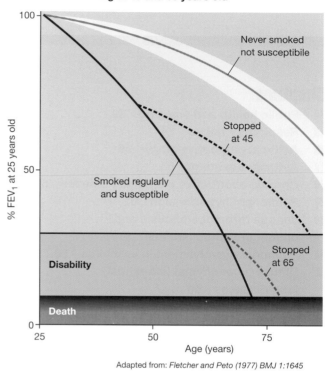

Adapted from: *Fletcher and Peto (1977) BMJ 1:1645*

Respiratory disease accounts for approximately 20% of all deaths in the UK. Acute infections (30.5%), progressive non-malignant disease (30.6%) and lung cancer (29.6%) are the main causes (Fig. 24a). Annually respiratory illness is responsible for approximately 850,000 hospital admissions, >30% of emergency medical admissions and 10% of hospital bed days. Chest disease varies geographically in relation to socioeconomic conditions with acute infectious illness, HIV-related disease and post-tuberculous bronchiectasis more frequent in developing countries and chronic obstructive pulmonary disease (COPD), cystic fibrosis and restrictive chest wall defects (e.g. obesity hypoventilation and muscular dystrophy) more common in the USA and Europe.

Factors associated with respiratory disease

1 *Smoking-related disease (SRD)* is recognized as the single greatest cause of preventable illness and mortality. It accounts for 5 million deaths/year worldwide and 114,000 deaths/year in the UK due to a wide variety of illness including lung or non-respiratory cancers (e.g. renal and bladder), COPD, ischaemic heart disease (IHD), peripheral vascular disease, stroke, pneumonia, interstitial lung disease, venous thromboembolism, diabetes, inflammatory bowel and peptic ulcer disease. In pregnancy smoking impedes fetal growth and increases the risk of obstructive airways disease in the child. Inhaled 'second-hand' or passive smoking increases lung cancer risk and is thought to cause approximately 12,000 deaths/year in the UK of which approximately 500 are due to workplace smoke exposure.

Tobacco smoke contains many potentially toxic gases including carbon monoxide, detected as carboxyhaemoglobin in the blood, and polycyclic aromatic hydrocarbons which cause gene mutations frequently found in primary lung cancers. Cigarette smoke accelerates normal age-related loss of lung function (Fig. 24b) and is the principal cause of COPD (Chapter 28). It also impairs epithelial ciliary function and mucociliary transport (Chapter 19), and stimulates goblet cell hyperplasia which contributes to the characteristic morning cough and excessive sputum expectoration experienced by regular smokers. Worldwide, 20 billion cigarettes are smoked by 2 billion individuals. Oral and other smoked tobacco products are also popular. However, recent legislation, smoking bans, changes in social attitude and taxation have significantly reduced the numbers of people smoking. Consequently, in many developed countries, the incidence of SRD is no longer rising (e.g. UK), or has fallen (e.g. USA). Sadly, increased smoking in developing societies, partly due to advertising, means that the current low levels of SRD in these countries are likely to rise.

- **COPD** will rank third in worldwide burden of disease by 2020. In the UK it affects approximately 14% of people over 35 years old (7–18% of men and 3–7% of women). However, COPD is often unrecognized, despite relatively severe disease, and only 0.9 of 3 million probable UK cases have been diagnosed. In the USA approximately 2 million people have emphysema and half have reduced exercise tolerance. COPD exacerbations are the commonest cause of emergency hospital admission (Fig. 24c), with an average hospital stay of 5 days, result in 24 million lost working days annually, account for approximately 13% of adult disability and cost the economy approximately £2 billion/year in the UK.
- **Lung cancer** (Chapter 42) is the commonest cause of cancer death in men and women in the USA and Europe. Smoking increases the risk by 30-fold compared to non-smokers (<1% lifetime risk) and is dependent on dose (i.e. number of cigarettes/day, depth of inhalation, years smoked), age of onset of smoking, ethnicity (e.g. greater in blacks), geographical area (e.g. Scotland and Kentucky) and pattern of smoking (i.e. quit periods reduce future risk). Age-standardized incidence rates are approximately $65/10^5$ for males and approximately $39/10^5$ for females in the UK and USA. In Europe, Hungary has the highest ($>100/10^5$) and Sweden the lowest ($<25/10^5$) incidence. Central Africa and south central Asia have the lowest lung cancer rates. In the UK, approximately 35,000 lung cancer deaths occur annually, and after prostate cancer, it is the second commonest cancer in men, causing approximately 22,000 new cases/year and third commonest in women after breast and bowel cancer, causing approximately 16,000 new cases/year.

2 **Environmental and social factors**. Air pollution (passive smoking), living conditions and poor sanitation increase susceptibility to acute infective diseases, asthma and hypersensitivity pneumonitis. Clean air initiatives, environmental legislation and socioeconomic programmes including better nutrition, access to clean water and education programmes (e.g. breast feeding and safe sex) have been beneficial.

- **Asthma** (Chapter 26) is the commonest respiratory disease in the UK, affecting 10–15% of the population, but there is considerable variation in worldwide prevalence, with highest levels in English-speaking countries. The cause of the recent increase in asthma incidence is unknown. Potential factors include dietary changes, improved standards of living, aeroallergens, environmental pollution, childhood infection and immunizations.

3 **Working conditions**. Protection against inhalation of mineral and organic dusts, chemicals and drugs have reduced susceptibility to occupational lung disease (e.g. coal workers' pneumoconiosis), work-related asthma and hypersensitivity pneumonitis (see Chapter 35).

Smoking cessation

In the UK, 24% of men and 23% of women smoke. However, smoking prevalence is highest in young adults (32% in 20–24 years old), manual occupations, socioeconomically deprived people and men of South Asian descent. Chinese and Indian women are least likely to smoke. Most smokers (>80%) start as teenagers and by 15 years of age 24% of girls and 16% of boys are regular smokers (average 42 cigarettes/week), despite it being illegal to sell tobacco to children. Factors associated with childhood smoking include parental smokers, one-parent families, poor academic progress and tobacco advertising.

Over two-thirds of smokers want to stop smoking. A third try every year. Successful smoking cessation reduces the risk of lung cancer by approximately 90%, but the risk is always higher than in lifelong non-smokers. The main barrier to smoking cessation is nicotine, which is highly addictive. Inhaled nicotine reaches the brain within 7–10 seconds of smoking a cigarette. It acts on brain nicotinic acetylcholine receptors (nAChR), which release neurotransmitters including noradrenaline (arousal, appetite reduction), serotonin (mood regulation), vasopressin (memory improvement), β-endorphin (anxiety reduction), and most importantly dopamine from the mesolimbic dopamine system or 'brain reward pathway' which elicits pleasure and is associated with the development of addictive behaviour. Smoking cessation results in physical and psychological withdrawal from the effects of these neurotransmitters and is associated with increased appetite and an average weight gain of 2 kg.

Management

Success of smoking cessation depends on both behavioural and pharmacological therapies. It is vital that the smoker is motivated to stop at the outset. To achieve sustained abstinence, the initial short-term nicotine craving is relieved with pharmacotherapy for 6–12 weeks, followed by ongoing intensive behaviour support.

a Behavioural strategies

All health professionals should address smoking cessation at every opportunity. Simple clinician counselling stimulates a quit attempt in 40% of smokers. Counselling includes the 5 As:

- **A**sk how much a person smokes (document pack years)
- **A**ssess risk of continued smoking and inform the patient
- **A**dvise how to stop smoking and what help is available
- **A**ssist with behavioural support or replacement therapy
- **A**rrange follow-up

Although brief counselling alone is only associated with quit rates of 1–3%, more intensive individual and group-counselling sessions with a 'quit date' can achieve abstinence in 20% at 1 year follow-up. Telephone follow-up, web-based support and multiple interviews – all improve cessation rates. Evidence for benefit with hypnosis or acupuncture is weak, but these are helpful after previous failed attempts.

b Pharmacotherapy

Nicotine replacement therapy (NRT) ameliorates nicotine withdrawal symptoms including insomnia, irritability, anger, anxiety, poor concentration and increased appetite. It is safe, even in patients with known cardiovascular diseases. Intensive behavioural support, combined with NRT, can achieve 1-year abstinence rates of 25% (compared to ~10% with usual care). Nicotine is available as transdermal patches, gum, sublingual tablets, nasal sprays and inhalers; all are equally effective. A patch raises baseline blood nicotine levels, but combined use of a second NRT (e.g. gums, lozenges, inhalers) to provide 'bursts of nicotine' helps overcome breakthrough urges, improving long-term success.

Antidepressants correct the low dopamine levels due to nicotine dependence. Smokers who are not depressed may also benefit from this approach. **Bupropion (Zyban)**, a dopamine uptake inhibitor, doubles normal quit rates. Combination with nicotine patches is not always beneficial. Bupropion is contraindicated in epilepsy and pregnancy. **Nortriptyline**, a tricyclic antidepressant, is an effective second-line agent.

Varenicline, a partial agonist of nAChR, reduces withdrawal cravings and decreases the reward effects of smoking. Twelve-week quit rates comparing varenicline, bupropion and placebo were 45, 30 and 18%, respectively, and at 12 months were 23, 16, and 9%, respectively. Varenicline is particularly effective when combined with intensive behavioural therapy.

25 Respiratory failure

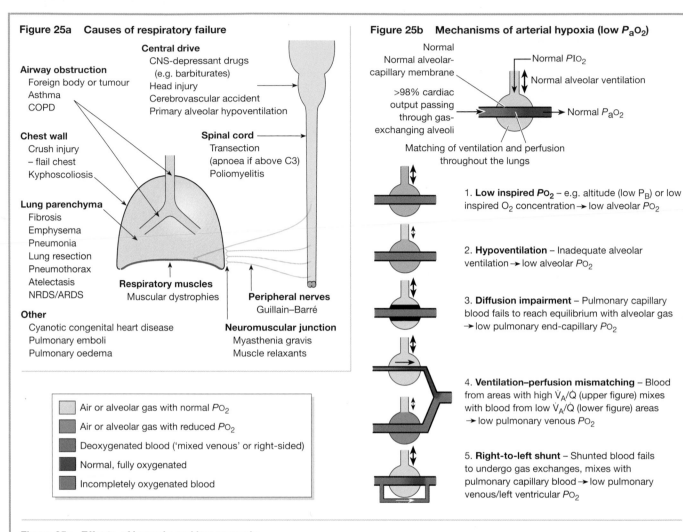

Figure 25a Causes of respiratory failure

Central drive
CNS-depressant drugs
(e.g. barbiturates)
Head injury
Cerebrovascular accident
Primary alveolar hypoventilation

Airway obstruction
Foreign body or tumour
Asthma
COPD

Chest wall
Crush injury
– flail chest
Kyphoscoliosis

Spinal cord
Transection
(apnoea if above C3)
Poliomyelitis

Lung parenchyma
Fibrosis
Emphysema
Pneumonia
Lung resection
Pneumothorax
Atelectasis
NRDS/ARDS

Respiratory muscles
Muscular dystrophies

Peripheral nerves
Guillain–Barré

Neuromuscular junction
Myasthenia gravis
Muscle relaxants

Other
Cyanotic congenital heart disease
Pulmonary emboli
Pulmonary oedema

Air or alveolar gas with normal P_{O_2}

Air or alveolar gas with reduced P_{O_2}

Deoxygenated blood ('mixed venous' or right-sided)

Normal, fully oxygenated

Incompletely oxygenated blood

Figure 25b Mechanisms of arterial hypoxia (low P_aO_2)

Normal
Normal alveolar-capillary membrane
>98% cardiac output passing through gas-exchanging alveoli
Matching of ventilation and perfusion throughout the lungs

Normal PI_{O_2}
Normal alveolar ventilation
Normal P_aO_2

1. **Low inspired P_{O_2}** – e.g. altitude (low P_B) or low inspired O_2 concentration → low alveolar P_{O_2}

2. **Hypoventilation** – Inadequate alveolar ventilation → low alveolar P_{O_2}

3. **Diffusion impairment** – Pulmonary capillary blood fails to reach equilibrium with alveolar gas → low pulmonary end-capillary P_{O_2}

4. **Ventilation–perfusion mismatching** – Blood from areas with high $\dot{V}_A/\dot{Q}$ (upper figure) mixes with blood from low $\dot{V}_A/\dot{Q}$ (lower figure) areas → low pulmonary venous P_{O_2}

5. **Right-to-left shunt** – Shunted blood fails to undergo gas exchanges, mixes with pulmonary capillary blood → low pulmonary venous/left ventricular P_{O_2}

Figure 25c Effects of hypoxia and hypercapnia

	Acute	Chronic—compensation and complications
Low P_aO_2 (hypoxaemia/ hypoxia)	**Impaired CNS function:** irritability, confusion, drowsiness, convulsions, coma, death **Central cyanosis** (not very sensitive; may be absent in anaemia) **Cardiac arrhythmias** **Hypoxic vasoconstriction*** of pulmonary vessels	**Erythropoietin** from hypoxic kidney → **polycythaemia** → ↑oxygen carriage despite low P_aO_2 but if excessive (haematocrit >55%) the ↑viscosity impairs tissue blood flow **Polycythaemia** → florid complexion; increased cyanosis **Pulmonary hypertension*** → right ventricular hypertrophy **Fluid retention/right heart failure (cor pulmonale*)** → peripheral oedema/ascites/↑jugular venous pressure/enlarged liver
High P_aCO_2 (hypercapnia)	**Low arterial pH** (respiratory acidosis) **Peripheral vasodilatation** → warm flushed skin, bounding pulse **Cerebral vasodilatation** → ↑intracranial pressure → headache, worse on waking if nocturnal ventilation↓ **Impaired CNS/muscle function:** irritability, confusion, somnolence, coma, tremor, myolonic jerks, hand flap **Cardiac arrhythmias**	**Renal compensation** (compensatory metabolic alkalosis) → ↑arterial [HCO_3^-] → arterial pH returned to near normal **Cerebrospinal fluid (CSF) compensation** → ↑CSF [HCO_3^-] → CSF pH returned to near normal → respiratory drive less at any given P_aCO_2 than in acute hypercapnia *Hypercapnia accentuates the vasoconstrictor effects of hypoxia on pulmonary blood vessels and therefore contributes to the development of cor pulmonale (see above)

Respiratory failure is usually said to exist when arterial P_{O_2} falls below 8 kPa (60 mmHg) when breathing air at sea level. In **type 1 respiratory failure**, the arterial hypoxia is accompanied by a normal or low arterial P_{CO_2}, whereas in **type 2 or ventilatory failure**, arterial P_{CO_2} is increased above 6.7 kPa (50 mmHg). Respiratory failure may be **acute** or **chronic**. In chronic respiratory failure, there are permanent abnormalities in blood gases, which typically worsen periodically (**acute on chronic**). This strict definition excludes some patients whose respiratory systems might otherwise be considered failing. Some patients have disabling **dyspnoea** (breathlessness) of respiratory origin but maintain an arterial P_{O_2} >8 kPa. Some of the many causes of respiratory failure are listed in Figure 25a. Symptoms and signs clearly depend on the underlying cause. Dyspnoea and **tachypnoea** (increased respiratory rate) will be prominent in severe asthma but absent in conditions with reduced central drive.

Mechanisms leading to hypoxia and hypercapnia

Of the five causes of hypoxaemia (Fig. 25b), only **hypoventilation** inevitably causes increased $P_{a}CO_2$.

$$P_{a}CO_2 \propto \frac{\dot{V}CO_2}{\dot{V}_A} \text{ (Chapter 9)}$$

If hypoxia is out of proportion to the hypercapnia and the **A–a P_{O_2} gradient** (Chapter 15) is increased, one of the other mechanisms (3–5 in Fig. 25b) must also be present. The primary effect of **right-to-left shunts** and **ventilation–perfusion mismatching** is to raise arterial CO_2 content, but this is usually corrected or overcorrected by a reflex increase in ventilation (Chapters 14 and 15).

Thickening of the alveolar–capillary membrane in lung fibrosis may give rise to **diffusion impairment**, preventing equilibration of pulmonary capillary blood with alveolar gas, especially in exercise, when time in the capillary is reduced. However, in many conditions thought to cause diffusion impairment, there is also substantial V_A/Q mismatching, and this is probably the main cause of the hypoxia.

Effects of hypoxia and hypercapnia

The direct effects of hypoxia and hypercapnia, together with the compensations and complications that occur in chronic respiratory failure, are shown in Figure 25c.

Although hypoxia usually offers the greatest threat to vital organs, hypercapnia and especially acidosis are also important and they often accentuate the adverse effects of each other. Hypoxia and hypercapnia are better tolerated when they develop slowly in chronic respiratory failure because of adaptations such as polycythaemia and compensatory metabolic alkalosis.

Cyanosis is a greyish-blue tinge seen when the microcirculation of a tissue contains a high concentration of deoxygenated haemoglobin. It may occur with impaired blood flow, for example, in the hands and feet in circulatory shock, when it is known as **peripheral cyanosis**. When the arterial blood contains more than about 1.5–2 g/dL of deoxygenated haemoglobin, the concentration in the microcirculation reaches the critical level for cyanosis to be observable even in well-perfused tissues. This occurs with an arterial saturation of about 85–90% if haemoglobin concentration is normal (150 g/L) and the resulting **central cyanosis** is visible in the tongue and mucous membranes of the mouth (tissues rarely affected by poor blood flow); as this requires a fall in $P_{a}O_2$ to 6.7–8 kPa (50–60 mmHg) from the normal sea level value of 13.3 kPa (100 mmHg), cyanosis is not very sensitive as an index of arterial hypoxia. It appears with a smaller fall in $P_{a}O_2$ and saturation in polycythaemic patients, whereas in severe anaemia central cyanosis may be impossible, as it would require a $P_{a}O_2$ incompatible with life.

Respiratory failure in asthma

Hypoxia in a severe asthma attack is primarily due to V_A/Q mismatching. $P_{a}CO_2$ usually falls as the attack worsens, because peripheral chemoreceptor and pulmonary receptor stimulation produce a reflex increase in ventilation despite the increased work of breathing. A raised or even apparently normal $P_{a}CO_2$ (e.g. 5.3 kPa, 40 mmHg) in a severely hypoxic asthma attack is a cause for concern, as it may indicate the onset of exhaustion and potentially life-threatening asthma.

Respiratory failure in chronic obstructive pulmonary disease

The clinical picture of severe chronic obstructive pulmonary disease (COPD) is variable (Chapter 28), but two extreme patterns – the **pink puffer** (dyspnoea, no cyanosis at rest) and the **blue bloater** (cyanosis at rest, cor pulmonale, oedema) – are recognized. The blue bloater is associated with type 2 respiratory failure. He or she has a chronically low $P_{a}O_2$ and high $P_{a}CO_2$, and these worsen with acute infections, which precipitate acute on chronic respiratory failure. Patients with chronic hypercapnia typically have a near-normal arterial pH owing to an efficient compensatory metabolic alkalosis via renal generation and retention of bicarbonate. During an acute exacerbation, $P_{a}CO_2$ may increase further and arterial pH then falls significantly, as renal adjustments are slow. Arterial pH can therefore indicate the proportions of acute and chronic hypercapnia. Patients with chronic hypercapnia are at risk of respiratory depression and a further, potentially fatal, increase in $P_{a}CO_2$ if given high inspired oxygen (Chapter 45). This may be due to loss of hypoxic drive in the presence of reduced CO_2 sensitivity, but other mechanisms may contribute to the rise in $P_{a}CO_2$, including increased V_A/Q mismatching by the removal of hypoxic vasoconstriction. As these patients are on the steep part of the oxyhaemoglobin dissociation curve, significant improvements in arterial oxygen content can usually be achieved by small increases in F_IO_2 (to 24% or 28%). The resulting small improvement in $P_{a}O_2$ does not cause respiratory depression (Chapter 13).

Management

All patients suspected of having respiratory failure will need arterial blood gas measurement, as the severity is difficult to assess clinically. A chest X-ray helps detect possible causes and aggravating factors such as pneumonia or pneumothorax. Other investigations, including lung function tests, will depend on the clinical situation and likely underlying disease. Management will include airway maintenance, clearance of secretions, oxygen therapy (Chapter 45) and in some cases mechanical ventilation (Chapter 44). Specific therapies, such as bronchodilators and antibiotics, are directed at the underlying cause or aggravating factors. Abnormalities in haemoglobin concentration, fluid balance and cardiac output should be treated to improve tissue oxygen delivery and increase mixed venous oxygen content, which in turn will also reduce the effects of any venous admixture on arterial oxygenation.

26 Asthma: pathophysiology

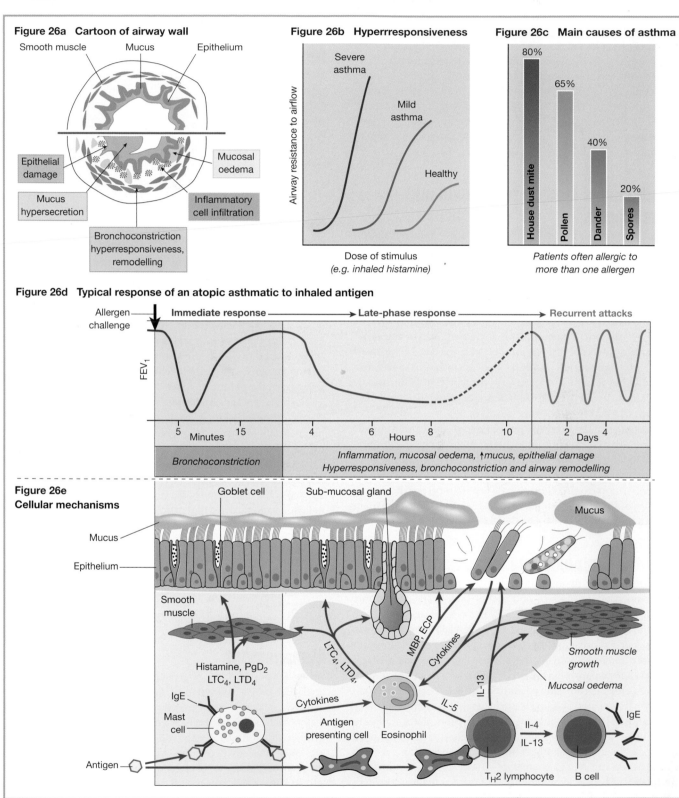

Figure 26a Cartoon of airway wall

Smooth muscle   Mucus   Epithelium

Epithelial damage

Mucus hypersecretion

Bronchoconstriction hyperresponsiveness, remodelling

Mucosal oedema

Inflammatory cell infiltration

Figure 26b Hyperrresponsiveness

Airway resistance to airflow

Severe asthma

Mild asthma

Healthy

Dose of stimulus (e.g. inhaled histamine)

Figure 26c Main causes of asthma

80% House dust mite
65% Pollen
40% Dander
20% Spores

Patients often allergic to more than one allergen

Figure 26d Typical response of an atopic asthmatic to inhaled antigen

Allergen challenge

Immediate response ————————→ **Late-phase response** ————————→ **Recurrent attacks**

FEV_1

5   15   Minutes
4   6   8   10   Hours
2   4   Days

Bronchoconstriction

*Inflammation, mucosal oedema, ↑mucus, epithelial damage
Hyperresponsiveness, bronchoconstriction and airway remodelling*

**Figure 26e
Cellular mechanisms**

Goblet cell   Sub-mucosal gland   Mucus

Mucus

Epithelium

Smooth muscle

Histamine, PgD_2
LTC_4, LTD_4

IgE

Mast cell

Antigen

LTC_4, LTD_4,

MBP, ECP

Cytokines

Cytokines

Antigen presenting cell   Eosinophil

IL-5

IL-13

Il-4
IL-13

T_H2 lymphocyte   B cell

Smooth muscle growth

Mucosal oedema

IgE

The Respiratory System at a Glance, Fourth Edition. Jeremy P.T. Ward. © Jeremy P.T. Ward. Published 2015 by John Wiley & Sons, Ltd.

Asthma is an inflammatory disorder of the airways. Patients suffer from episodes of cough, wheezing, chest tightness and/or dyspnoea (breathlessness), which are often worse at night or early in the morning. Asthma can be defined as 'a chronic inflammatory disorder characterized by increased responsiveness of the bronchi to various innocuous stimuli, manifested by widespread and variable airway narrowing that varies in severity either spontaneously or with treatment'. The major characteristics of asthma are (Fig. 26a):

1 Narrowing of the airways and impeded airflow, commonly reversible spontaneously or following treatment.
2 Non-specific airway **hyperresponsiveness** to a range of normally innocuous stimuli (e.g. cold air, irritants and pollutants) and airway spasmogens leading to bronchoconstriction (Fig. 26b).
3 Increased mucosal inflammation and recruitment of **inflammatory cells** (eosinophils, mast cells, neutrophils, T lymphocytes) to the airways.

There is also **hypersecretion of mucus**, which can lead to blockage of airways with **mucus plugs**, and swelling of mucosa due to inflammation-associated vascular leak and consequent **oedema** of the airway wall, all of which further limit airflow. Damage to the epithelium (**epithelial shedding**) is reflected by whorls of epithelial cells (Curschmann's spirals) in the mucus, which also contains eosinophil cell membranes (Charcot–Leyden crystals). In chronic asthma **remodelling of the airway wall** structure occurs, including increased bronchial smooth muscle content. This causes irreversible narrowing of the airways and limits the effectiveness of bronchodilators.

Prevalence

Asthma is increasing in prevalence, particularly in the Western world, where more than 5% of the population may be symptomatic and receiving treatment. There has been a concomitant increase in mortality, despite improved treatment. In the UK, one in seven of the population has allergic disease and over 9 million people will have wheezed in the last year. The number of teenagers with asthma has nearly doubled over the last 12 years. Asthma is least common in the Far East and most common in the UK, Australia and New Zealand. There is some correlation with Westernized lifestyles; the "**hygiene hypothesis**" proposes that lack of early exposure to pathogens and helminths predisposes to allergies. Children brought up on farms have a reduced prevalence of allergy and asthma. Many factors can precipitate an asthma attack or worsen symptoms, including exposure to specific **antigens**, **tobacco smoke** and **exhaust fumes**, and **emotional stress**. Exercise (**exercised-induced asthma**) and inhalation of cold air often precipitate wheezing in asthmatics, probably via drying and cooling of the bronchial epithelium, and is common in children. Certain **viral infections** (rhinovirus, parainfluenza, respiratory syncytial virus) are associated with asthma attacks. There may also be a genetic component to asthma. Importantly, 20% of the working population may be susceptible to **occupational asthma** due to their working environment (Chapter 35).

Classification

Asthma can be classified as **extrinsic**, having a definite external cause, and **intrinsic**, where no external cause can be identified. Extrinsic asthma commonly occurs as a result of an allergic response (Chapter 20), with development of **IgE antibodies** to specific antigens (**allergic** or **atopic asthma**), and tends to start in childhood with symptoms becoming less severe with age; approximately 80% of asthmatics are atopic. Intrinsic asthma generally appears in adults and is **IgE independent**.

Atopic asthma

Individuals who readily produce IgE to common antigens are prone to allergic asthma. Major antigens include proteins in fecal pellets from **house dust mite** (*Dermatophagoides pteronyssinus*; **DerP**) – the most common cause of asthma worldwide – grass and tree **pollen**, dander (skin flakes) from **domestic pets** and **fungal spores** (Fig. 26c). Genetic factors, early environment and maternal smoking in pregnancy may predispose to raised IgE levels and later development of asthma and airway hyper-responsiveness.

Inhalation of allergens by atopic individuals initiates an **immediate response** (bronchoconstriction) that usually subsides within 2 hours (Fig. 26d) and is reversible with bronchodilators such as β_2-adrenoceptor agonists (Chapter 27). This is often followed 3–12 hours later by a **late-phase response** with bronchoconstriction, airway inflammation and oedema, and hyper-responsiveness (Fig. 26d), which is less susceptible to bronchodilators. Some materials (e.g. **isocyanates**) cause only an **isolated late phase**. Increased hyper-responsiveness may promote **recurrent asthma attacks** over several days.

The immediate response is an example of **type I hypersensitivity**. It is caused by antigen/IgE-induced **mast cell degranulation** and release of **histamine, prostaglandin D_2** (PgD_2) and **leukotriene C_4 and D_4** (LTC_4, LTD_4); these cause bronchoconstriction, increased mucus production and vascular leak (Fig. 26e). The late phase (an example of **type IV** or **cell-based hypersensitivity**) is primarily due to inflammation. Allergic inflammation characteristically involves T_H2 **lymphocytes** (Chapter 20). Asthma is therefore often described as a T_H2-driven disease, and may involve an imbalance between T_H1 and T_H2 pathways. On activation by **antigen presenting cells**, T_H2 cells release specific **cytokines** (cellular mediators) including interleukin-5 (IL-5), which promotes **eosinophil** proliferation, maturation and survival, and IL-4 and IL-13 which stimulate B cell class switching and production of IgE (Chapter 20). IL-13 plays a key role in the pathology of asthma, as it also stimulates epithelial cells (also airway smooth muscle cells and fibroblasts), causing release of multiple mediators and consequent mucus overproduction, airway hyper-responsiveness and recruitment of immune cells including eosinophils (Fig. 26e).

Eosinophils are present in large numbers in asthmatic bronchi, and release **leukotrienes, major basic protein** (MBP) and **eosinophil cationic protein** (ECP). MBP and ECP contribute to epithelial cell damage and activation, causing further release of mediators, increased permeability to allergens, and exposure of C-fibre sensory nerves which release proinflammatory tachykinins.

Drug-associated asthma

Aspirin and other non-steroidal anti-inflammatory drugs (NSAIDs) promote asthmatic attacks in 5% of asthmatics. They inhibit the cyclooxygenase (COX) pathway that synthesizes prostaglandins and shift arachidonic acid metabolism from COX towards the lipoxygenase pathway and production of leukotrienes. Aspirin-induced asthma is partially reversed by antileukotriene therapy (Chapter 27).

The bronchi have little sympathetic innervation, but circulating adrenaline acting via β_2-adrenoceptors on smooth muscle causes bronchodilatation. Consequently β-adrenoceptor antagonists can cause bronchoconstriction in asthmatics. This may even occur with nominally β_1-selective drugs, and their use for cardiovascular disease should be avoided in asthmatics.

27 Asthma: treatment

Figure 27a Step-wise approach to asthma therapy (adult)

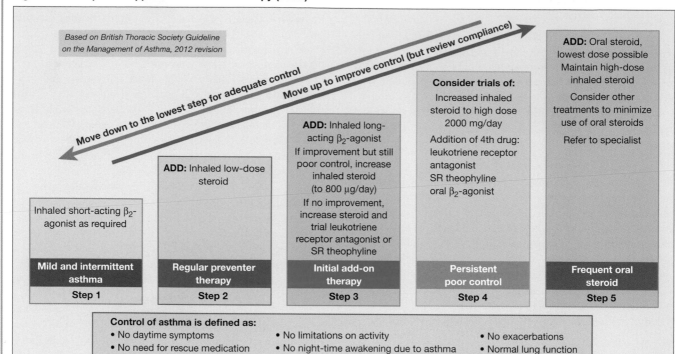

Based on British Thoracic Society Guideline on the Management of Asthma, 2012 revision

Move down to the lowest step for adequate control

Move up to improve control (but review compliance)

Inhaled short-acting β₂-agonist as required

Mild and intermittent asthma

Step 1

ADD: Inhaled low-dose steroid

Regular preventer therapy

Step 2

ADD: Inhaled long-acting β₂-agonist
If improvement but still poor control, increase inhaled steroid (to 800 µg/day)
If no improvement, increase steroid and trial leukotriene receptor antagonist or SR theophyline

Initial add-on therapy

Step 3

Consider trials of:
Increased inhaled steroid to high dose 2000 mg/day
Addition of 4th drug: leukotriene receptor antagonist
SR theophyline
oral β₂-agonist

Persistent poor control

Step 4

ADD: Oral steroid, lowest dose possible
Maintain high-dose inhaled steroid
Consider other treatments to minimize use of oral steroids
Refer to specialist

Frequent oral steroid

Step 5

Control of asthma is defined as:
- No daytime symptoms
- No need for rescue medication
- No limitations on activity
- No night-time awakening due to asthma
- No exacerbations
- Normal lung function

Figure 27b Most common drug classes used in asthma

Type	Route and example	Effect	Adverse effects
β₂–agonist (adrenoreceptor agonists)	**Inhaled, oral, intravenous (IV)** Short-acting: *salbutamol (albuterol)* Long-acting: *salmeterol, formoterol*	**Bronchodilators** May stabilize mast cells *(increase cAMP)*	Muscle tremor (most common) Tachycardia, palpitations (high dose)
Corticosteroids	**Inhaled:** *Beclometasone, fluticasone* **Oral:** *Prednisolene* **IV:** *Hydrocortisone*	**Anti-inflammatory** *(Suppress activation of inflammatory genes)*	**Inhaled:** oral candidiasis, cough, hoarseness **Oral/high dose:** Retarded growth, water retention, osteoporosis, hypertension, weight gain, eye problems, diabetes, psychosis
Xanthines	**Oral, IV:** *Theophylline, aminophylline* *Slow release (SR) formulations*	**Bronchodilators** Some anti-inflammatory action *(increase cAMP)*	Headache, nausea, diuresis, cardiac arrhythmias, vomiting, epilepsy; many drug interactions affect xanthine plasma levels
Muscarinic receptor antagonists	**Inhaled:** *Ipratropium bromide*	**Bronchodilators** Reduce mucus secretion *(block cholinergic effects)*	Rare, bitter taste
Leukotriene receptor antagonists (LTRA)	**Oral:** *Montelukast, zafirlukast*	**Bronchodilators, anti-inflammatory** May reduce mucosal oedema *(block action of LTC_4, LTD_4)*	Rare, liver problems

Figure 27c Pressurized metered dose inhaler

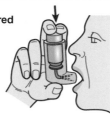

- Remove the cap and shake the inhaler
- Tilt the head back slightly and exhale
- Position the inhaler in the mouth (or preferably just in front of the open mouth)
- During a slow inspiration, press down the inhaler to release the medication
- Continue inhalation to full inspiration
- Hold breath for 10 seconds
- Actuate only one puff per inhalation

The Respiratory System at a Glance, Fourth Edition. Jeremy P.T. Ward. © Jeremy P.T. Ward. Published 2015 by John Wiley & Sons, Ltd.

Management of asthma should encompass assessment of severity and efficacy of therapy, identification and removal of precipitating factors, therapy to reverse bronchoconstriction and inflammation, patient and family participation and education. Diagnosis is determined on the basis of a characteristic pattern of signs and symptoms in the absence of alternative explanations.

Assessment

Lung function: Primary assessment is with spirometry. Asthma is probable when inhaled bronchodilators cause more than 15% improvement in forced expiratory volume in 1 second (FEV_1) or peak expiratory flow rate (PEFR) (Chapter 22). The absence of improvement does not rule out asthma – the patient could be in remission and chronic severe asthma is poorly reversible. Airway resistance is least at midday and greatest at 3–4 AM. Serial measurements of PEFR in the morning, midday and on retiring are useful for identifying the enhanced variation in airflow limitation characteristic of asthma and for assessing response to therapy over time. Poorly controlled asthma shows a characteristic morning fall in PEFR (**morning dipping**). Occupational asthma is suggested when PEFR improves after a break from work. Lung function tests are often coupled with exercise tests in children, who often exhibit exercise-induced asthma.

Bronchial provocation tests can determine **hyperresponsiveness** (Chapter 26) when asthma is suspected but spirometry is not diagnostic. Patients inhale increasing doses of histamine or methacholine (acetylcholine analogue) until FEV_1 declines by 20%. The dose at which this occurs ($PD_{20}FEV_1$) is greatly reduced in asthmatics, who are always hyperresponsive (Fig. 26b).

Skin prick tests identify extrinsic factors. Development of a wheal around the prick site indicates allergen sensitivity. Exposure to identified allergens should be minimized (e.g. replacement of furnishings to reduce house dust mite, removal of pets). Only 50% of patients with occupational asthma are cured by avoidance of precipitating factors.

Therapy

The goal is long-term control, and all patients except those with the mildest symptoms should receive anti-inflammatory drugs as well as bronchodilators. International guidelines favour **step-wise treatment regimens** (Fig. 27a). Asthma therapy is centred on **inhaled** compounds (Fig. 27b), which maximize bronchial delivery while minimizing systemic side effects. Metered dose inhalers (**MDI**) are the commonest delivery system, although only approximately 15–20% of the dose may reach the lungs (Fig. 27c); this can be improved by use of spacers. Asthma drugs are often called **relievers**, bronchodilators that relieve acute symptoms, or **preventers**, prophylactic and anti-inflammatory drugs that relieve chronic symptoms and hyperresponsiveness; some have both properties. Histamine antagonists have not proved useful in asthma.

Short-acting β_2-adrenoceptor agonists (e.g. salbutamol) are rapid and powerful bronchodilators (relievers) and are first choice for alleviating acute symptoms. They activate adenylate cyclase to increase cyclic adenosine monophosphate (cAMP). They also reduce activation of mast cells. **Long-acting β_2-agonists** (LABA, e.g. salmeterol) are used prophylactically, but must only be used for patients already on steroids (see below). Long-term use of β_2-agonists is associated with reduced effectiveness (**tolerance**).

Corticosteroids are the most important anti-inflammatory (preventer) drugs, and suppress inflammatory gene activation. Steroids reduce eosinophil numbers and activity of macrophages and lymphocytes. **Inhaled steroids** (e.g. beclomethasone, fluticasone) are the mainstay of asthma therapy. Low doses are safe but can cause oral candidiasis (5%) and hoarseness. Growth may be retarded in children receiving high-dose inhaled corticosteroids. **Oral corticosteroids** such as prednisolone may be required in patients whose asthma cannot be controlled by inhaled steroids, but the danger of adverse effects is much greater. **Combination therapies** containing both steroid and LABA are commonly used for moderate/severe asthmatics.

Muscarinic receptor antagonists (e.g. ipratropium) block the effects of acetylcholine from parasympathetic nerves to smooth muscle and mucus glands. They are moderately effective bronchodilators and reduce mucus secretion. They are slower and less effective than β_2-agonists, and more useful against irritant than allergen-induced responses.

Xanthines (e.g. theophylline, aminophylline) have bronchodilatory and some anti-inflammatory actions and are taken orally. They inhibit phosphodiesterases that break down cAMP. Limitations include numerous side effects and a narrow therapeutic range; these are partially overcome by slow-release (SR) preparations. Used as second-line drugs in asthma, particularly when β_2-agonists are ineffective at controlling symptoms and in steroid-resistant asthma.

Leukotriene receptor antagonists (LTRAs; e.g. montelukast) block the cysLT receptor (LTC_4/D_4), and are taken orally as a prophylactic. They have relatively long-lasting bronchodilator and anti-inflammatory effects, and are particular effective for exercise-induced asthma and asthma associated with allergic rhinitis. They are also effective in aspirin-sensitive asthma, indicating the role leukotrienes have in this condition (Chapter 26). LTRAs may improve lung function in mild and moderate asthmatics, but greatest benefits may be for severe asthmatics taking steroids.

Cromones (sodium cromoglycate, nedocromil) inhibit activation of mast cells and eosinophils, and may suppress sensory nerves and release of neuropeptides (Chapter 26). They are only effective prophylactically. Use has declined as they are less effective and more expensive than modern low-dose steroids, but are useful when steroids cannot be used.

Recombinant anti-IgE antibody (omalizumab) has been shown to be effective in moderate to severe allergic asthma, by reducing levels of antigen-specific IgE. Promising results have been obtained in trials of anti-cytokine antibodies (e.g. anti-IL-13, anti-IL-5). All require specialist treatment centres.

Bronchial thermoplasty uses heat to reduce smooth muscle mass and function in medium airways, and has been used successfully in severe uncontrolled asthmatics.

Poorly controlled asthma is often related to poor compliance with treatment regimens – for example, due to peer pressure in children. Poor inhaler techniques are common. Compliance may also be poor when asthma is apparently controlled, so patients stop preventer therapies (e.g. steroids) because they are 'cured'. Patient education and training are therefore key to asthma therapy.

Severe uncontrolled asthma

Requires immediate treatment and hospitalization. **Indications:** inability to complete sentences ('telegraph speaking'), high respiratory rate, tachycardia, PEFR less than 50% predicted. Becomes **life-threatening** with one or more of: PEFR less than 33% predicted, hypoxaemia, hypercapnia, silent chest, exhaustion. **Treatment:** immediate nebulized β_2-agonists +/− ipratropium delivered in oxygen and intravenous steroids, with subsequent oral steroids. In unresolving cases, intravenous β_2-agonists or xanthines and ventilation may be required.

28 Chronic obstructive pulmonary disease

Figure 28a Risk factors for COPD

- Smoking
- Age >50 years old; prevalence ~5–10%
- Male gender
- Childhood chest infections
- Airways hyperreactivity
  – asthma/atopy
- Low socioeconomic status
  α1-Antitrypsin deficiency
- Heavy metal exposure
  – cadmium
- Atmospheric pollution

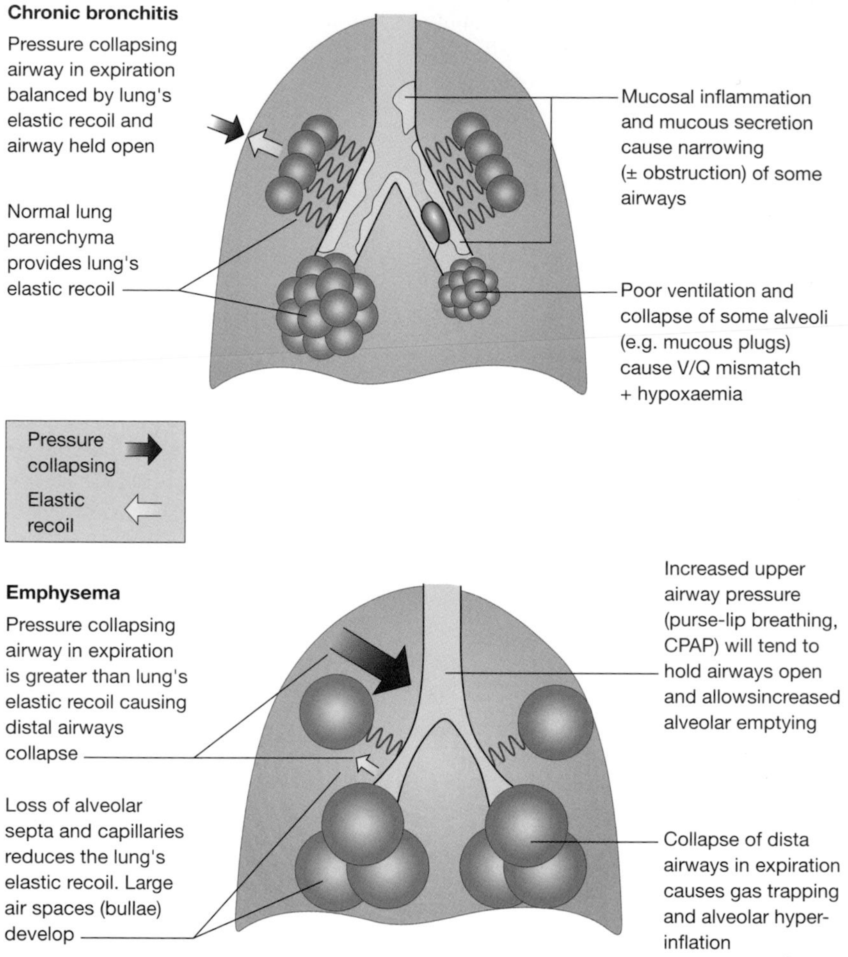

Figure 28c Spirometry. FEV$_1$/FVC ratio decreases in COPD

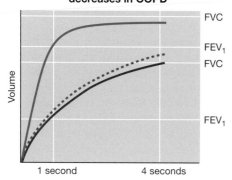

Normal ——
FEV$_1$/FVC = >0.8

COPD ——
FEV$_1$/FVC = <0.8

COPD ·······
Irreversible with bronchodilators
<15% increase in FEV$_1$

Figure 28b Pathophysiology of chronic bronchitis and emphysema

Chronic bronchitis

Pressure collapsing airway in expiration balanced by lung's elastic recoil and airway held open

Normal lung parenchyma provides lung's elastic recoil

Mucosal inflammation and mucous secretion cause narrowing (± obstruction) of some airways

Poor ventilation and collapse of some alveoli (e.g. mucous plugs) cause V/Q mismatch + hypoxaemia

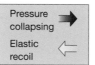

Pressure collapsing ➡

Elastic recoil ⬅

Emphysema

Pressure collapsing airway in expiration is greater than lung's elastic recoil causing distal airways collapse

Loss of alveolar septa and capillaries reduces the lung's elastic recoil. Large air spaces (bullae) develop

Increased upper airway pressure (purse-lip breathing, CPAP) will tend to hold airways open and allows increased alveolar emptying

Collapse of distal airways in expiration causes gas trapping and alveolar hyper-inflation

Figure 28d Typical signs and symptoms of COPD

Chronic bronchitis	Emphysema
Chronic cough, producing sputum Hypoventilation, little respiratory effort Cyanosis, hypoxaemia with secondary polycythaemia CO$_2$ retention/chronic hypercapnia – *leading to peripheral vasodilatation and bounding pulse* Oedema Cor pulmonale **Normal** lung volumes, D$_L$CO, lung compliance	Chronic breathlessness (dyspnoea) Cyanosis unusual; normoxic at rest, hypoxic on exercise Barrel chest (hyperinflation), underweight Rarely exhibit oedema or cor pulmonale **Increased** TLC, RV, lung compliance **Reduced** D$_L$CO
Note: Most patients may present with both chronic bronchitis and emphysema	

The Respiratory System at a Glance, Fourth Edition. Jeremy P.T. Ward. © Jeremy P.T. Ward. Published 2015 by John Wiley & Sons, Ltd.

Chronic obstructive pulmonary disease (COPD) is characterized by *persistent* airflow obstruction, hyperinflation and mucus hypersecretion, and is usually progressive and associated with chronic airway inflammation. COPD encompasses **chronic bronchitis** and **emphysema**, which often present together, but neither necessarily lead to airflow limitation. Smoking and other risk factors (Fig. 28a) accelerate the normal age-related decline in lung function (Chapter 24), and cause chronic respiratory symptoms interposed with intermittent **acute exacerbations**, eventually leading to disability and **respiratory failure** (Chapter 25). Chronic hypoxaemia can lead to **pulmonary hypertension** (Chapter 29). Asthma is not classified as COPD as the airflow obstruction is *reversible* (Chapters 26 and 27).

Diagnosis and pathophysiology

COPD is diagnosed by airflow obstruction indicated by a **reduced FEV_1/FVC ratio** of less than 0.7, which is irreversible (<15% increase in FEV_1) with bronchodilator or steroid therapy (Fig. 28c; Chapter 22). Restrictive lung disease (e.g. fibrosis) should be excluded. Patients with COPD exhibit **dyspnoea** (breathlessness) at rest or on exertion. Many smokers have lung function abnormalities that predate symptoms, which may be prevented by early smoking cessation.

Chronic bronchitis is associated with airways obstruction caused by **chronic mucosal inflammation**, **mucous gland hypertrophy** and **mucus hypersecretion**, coupled with **bronchospasm** (Fig. 28b). It is defined by daily morning cough and excessive mucus production for 3 months in 2 successive years, in the absence of airway tumour, acute/chronic infection or uncontrolled cardiac disease. Most patients have normal total lung capacity (TLC), functional residual capacity (FRC), residual volume (RV), D_LCO (diffusing capacity) and static lung compliance (Chapter 22). Patients with advanced chronic bronchitis have reduced respiratory drive and **CO_2 retention**, which is associated with bounding pulse, vasodilatation, confusion, headache, flapping tremor and papilloedema. **Hypoxaemia** is mostly due to V_A/Q mismatch (Fig. 28b; Chapter 15), and leads to **polycythaemia** (increased red cells) and **increased pulmonary artery pressure** (pulmonary hypertension) due to **hypoxic pulmonary vasoconstriction**. The resulting impairment of function of the right side of the heart leads to renal fluid retention, raised central venous pressure and **peripheral oedema**, subsequently leading to **cor pulmonale** (fluid retention/heart failure secondary to lung disease). Pulmonary hypertension is potentiated by extensive capillary loss in late disease. There are no radiographical signs diagnostic for chronic bronchitis.

Emphysema is caused by progressive destruction of alveolar septa and capillaries, leading to development of **enlarged airways and airspaces** (bullae), decreased lung elastic recoil and increased airway collapsibility. Airway obstruction is caused by collapse of distal airways during expiration due to loss of elastic radial traction present in the normal lung (Fig. 28b). The resulting **hyperinflation** enhances expiratory airflow, but inspiratory muscles work at a mechanical disadvantage. The pathophysiology of emphysema may involve an imbalance between inflammatory cell proteases and antiprotease defences (Chapters 19 and 20). Centrilobular emphysema is associated with cigarette smoking and predominantly involves the upper lung zones. Panacinar emphysema is associated with **α_1-antitrypsin deficiency** (Chapter 19) and predominantly involves the lower lung zones. Patients with emphysema typically have airflow obstruction with elevated TLC, FRC and RV, reduced D_LCO and increased static lung compliance. Such patients tend to be breathless and tachypnoeic (fast respiratory rate) at rest, with signs of hyperinflation and malnutrition including **barrel chest** and thin body, use of accessory respiratory muscles and **purse-lipped breathing**. The latter increases pressure in the upper airways and thus limits distal airway collapse. Auscultation reveals distant breath sounds with a prolonged expiratory wheeze. Blood gases are normal at rest, with marked O_2 desaturation during exertion. Radiographically, emphysema may appear as hyperinflated lungs with a large retrosternal airspace and flat diaphragms. When the condition is advanced, there may be areas with a lack of vascularity or visualization of bullae. High-resolution computed tomography (CT) is useful to demonstrate enlarged airspaces and air trapping.

Management

Treatment can slow, but not reverse, disease progression, ease chronic symptoms and prevent acute exacerbations. Smoking cessation is critical, and all COPD patients benefit from regular exercise. Therapy should be based on the GOLD (Global Initiative for Chronic Obstructive Lung Disease) guidelines.

Pharmacological therapy is similar to that for asthma (Chapter 27). Bronchodilators are central for managing symptoms: Short-acting inhaled **β_2-agonists** (e.g. salbutamol) and **anticholinergics** (e.g. ipratropium) improve symptoms and lung function, and have additive effects when combined. **Long-acting** β_2-agonists (LABA, e.g. salmeterol) and anticholinergics (LAMA, e.g. tiotropium) give more sustained relief and reduce exacerbations in more severe disease. **Inhaled corticosteroids** may be useful in severe disease (FEV_1 <50% predicted) and provide additional benefits in combination with LABA and LAMA. However, there is increased risk of pneumonia. Long-term oral corticosteroids are not recommended. Patients producing viscous sputum may benefit from **mucolytics**.

Pulmonary rehabilitation strengthens respiratory muscles and improves quality of life and exercise tolerance while reducing hospitalizations, but has no effect on lung function. **O_2 therapy** prolongs life in patients with resting daytime hypoxaemia by slowing progression of cor pulmonale. O_2 should be utilized as much as possible, as benefit increases with use. Patients with nocturnal or exercise desaturation benefit from supplemental O_2 at night or during exercise. In **α_1-antitrypsin deficiency**, replacement therapy can increase plasma and lung antiprotease levels; however, the benefits on lung function and survival are controversial. Surgical **lung volume reduction** or **transplantation** may be indicated in advanced COPD for carefully selected patients.

Prevention of acute COPD exacerbations includes pneumococcal and influenza vaccination. Patients with any combination of increased dyspnoea, increased sputum or purulent sputum benefit from antibiotics targeted against common respiratory pathogens (e.g. *Haemophilus influenzae*). Short courses of oral corticosteroids may improve lung function and hasten recovery in patients with acute exacerbations.

Overall prognosis for COPD patients is dependent on the severity of airflow obstruction. Patients with a FEV_1 less than 0.8 L have a yearly mortality of approximately 25%. Patients with cor pulmonale, hypercapnia, ongoing cigarette smoking and weight loss have a worse prognosis. Death usually occurs from infection, acute respiratory failure, pulmonary embolus or cardiac arrhythmia.

29 Pulmonary hypertension

Figure 29a Dana Point (2008) classification of pulmonary hypertension

Group 1: Pulmonary arterial hypertension (PAH)
1.1 Idiopathic (iPAH)
1.2 Heritable (hPAH)
1.3 Drug- and toxin-induced
1.4 Associated with (aPAH)
1.4.1 Connective tissue disease (e.g. systemic sclerosis)
1.4.2 HIV infection
1.4.3 Portal hypertension
1.4.4 Congenital heart disease
1.4.5 Schistosomiasis
1.4.6 Chronic haemolytic anaemia
1.5 Persistent pulmonary hypertension of the newborn

Group 1': PH associated with pulmonary veno-occlusive disease and/or pulmonary capillary haemangiomatosis

Group 2: PH caused by left heart disease
2.1 Systolic dysfunction
2.2 Diastolic dysfunction
2.3 Valvular disease

Group 3: PH caused by lung disease and/or hypoxia
3.1 Chronic obstructive pulmonary disease
3.2 Interstitial lung disease
3.3 Other pulmonary diseases with a mixed restrictive and obstructive pattern
3.4 Sleep-disordered breathing
3.5 Alveolar hypoventilation disorders
3.6 Chronic exposure to high altitude
3.7 Developmental abnormalities

Group 4: Chronic thromboembolic PH (CETPH)

Group 5: PH with unclear multifactorial mechanisms
5.1 Haematological disorders
5.2 Systemic disorders (e.g. sarcoidosis, vasculitis)
5.3 Metabolic disorders (e.g. glycogen storage disease)
5.4 Others (e.g. obstruction of PA by a tumour, chronic renal failure)

Figure 29b Pathogenesis of pulmonary hypertension by group

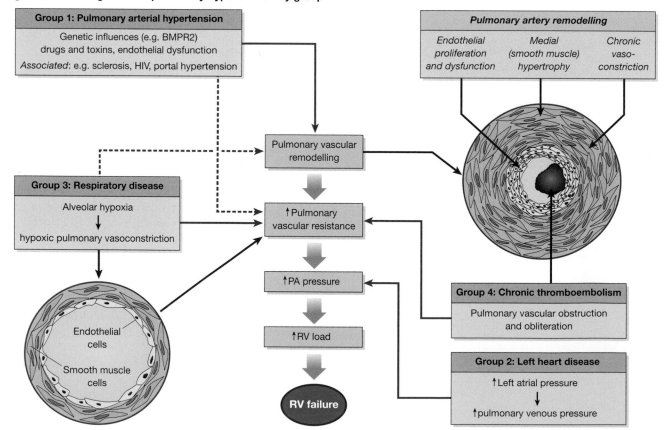

The Respiratory System at a Glance, Fourth Edition. Jeremy P.T. Ward. © Jeremy P.T. Ward. Published 2015 by John Wiley & Sons, Ltd.

Pulmonary hypertension (PH) is defined as a mean pulmonary artery (PA) pressure of more than **25 mmHg** at rest or more than **30 mmHg** during exercise (normal value ~14 mmHg mean). The rise in PA pressure can be due to increases in **pulmonary vascular resistance** (e.g. hypoxia and embolism), pulmonary blood flow or pulmonary venous pressure (e.g. left heart failure). PH is most commonly secondary to another condition; more rarely it is due to a disorder of the pulmonary circulation itself. The Dana Point (2008) classification of PH is shown in Figure 29a.

Types of pulmonary hypertension

Group 1, Pulmonary arterial hypertension (PAH): includes idiopathic (iPAH) and heritable PAH (hPAH), PAH associated with other conditions (aPAH), and persistent PH of the newborn. iPAH is rare (1–2 per million population) and its pathogenesis unclear, although both iPAH and hPAH are associated with reduced expression of **bone morphogenetic protein receptor type 2** (BMPR2). Genetic abnormalities, in particular related to BMPR2 and serotonin transporters, may predispose patients to PAH, but although some cases are clearly **familial** with autosomal dominant inheritance (hPAH), others are **sporadic** with no family history. iPAH is more common in women than men (ratio 2:1) and most prevalent between 20 and 40 years of age. Certain appetite-suppressant drugs affecting serotonin (e.g. fenfluramine) are associated with greatly increased risk. Remodelling of pulmonary arterioles is characteristic of PAH, although a component of arterial vasospasm is suggested by the effect of vasodilators (Fig. 29b). Conditions associated with PAH but where no causal relationship has been determined (aPAH) include collagen vascular disease, HIV infection and hepatic portal hypertension (Fig. 29a).

Groups 2–5 encompass PH caused by other disorders. **Group 2, Secondary to left heart disease:** increased left atrial (LA) pressure due to left ventricular dysfunction as in **congestive heart failure**, leads to elevation of PA pressure by increasing back-pressure through the lungs. **Mitral insufficiency** or **stenosis** may also increase PA pressure enough to cause hypertension. **Group 3, Secondary to respiratory disease:** due to hypoxaemia which causes small pulmonary arteries to constrict (**hypoxic pulmonary vasoconstriction**). Any condition leading to hypoxia can cause PH, including COPD (Chapter 28), sleep-disordered breathing (Chapter 46) and exposure to altitude (Chapter 16). Also associated with vascular remodelling, but much less severe than for PAH (Fig. 29b). **Group 4, Secondary to thrombotic disease:** chronic **thromboembolism** causes PH by mechanical obstruction of the proximal or distal pulmonary arteries. In acute thromboembolism, a component of vasospasm is also present, as the platelet-rich embolus releases vasoactive mediators such as thromboxane and serotonin. **Group 5, Multi-factorial, unclear mechanisms:** caused by heterogeneous conditions such as sarcoidosis, vasculitis, metabolic disorders, obstruction by tumours and others.

Clinical features

Development of PH can substantially increase morbidity and mortality. The prognosis for COPD patients with PH is much worse, with a 5-year survival for of less than 10% if PA pressure is more than 45 mmHg compared with more than 90% with PA pressure less than 25 mmHg. Mean survival without treatment in iPAH is 2 years. Patients usually die from **progressive right-sided heart failure**. Chronic PH can lead to pulmonary vascular remodelling and thickening of the pulmonary vasculature, reducing the efficacy of vasodilators. PH is generally slow to develop and presents with non-specific symptoms, including dyspnoea on exertion, shortness of breath, palpitations, chest pain, light-headedness and syncope. Signs are difficult to elicit early and may only include an increased pulmonic component of the second heart sound. With more severe hypertension, **right ventricular dysfunction** will be apparent, including jugular venous distension, right ventricular heave, pedal oedema and hepatic enlargement. Detection of PH requires a high index of suspicion, because signs and symptoms are non-specific and the diagnosis requires further testing; there is significant underdiagnosis.

Diagnosis

Evaluation of patients with suspected PH begins with **echocardiography**, allowing calculation of right ventricular systolic pressure and visualization of left atrium (LA), mitral valve, right ventricle and congenital abnormalities. If PH is found in conjunction with an enlarged LA, it is most likely due to either left ventricular or mitral disease. Chest radiology, pulmonary function testing and measurement of arterial oxygen allow detection of parenchymal disease or hypoxia. In the absence of LA enlargement or pulmonary parenchymal disease, further evaluation of pulmonary arteries is necessary. Ventilation/perfusion scanning is most useful to demonstrate chronic thromboemboli (Chapter 30). **Right heart catheterization** is the definitive test for the assessment of PH, as PA pressure can be measured directly and LA pressure estimated from the pulmonary capillary wedge pressure. Patients with PH without an elevated LA pressure and no apparent pulmonary venous, lung parenchymal, chronic thromboemboli or congenital heart disease are assumed to have PAH.

Management

Therapy in most patients is directed at the underlying abnormality, to relieve right ventricular strain and prevent right-sided heart failure. Hypoxaemic patients with COPD benefit from O_2 therapy to diminish hypoxic vasoconstriction. Patients with **thromboembolic disease** (Chapter 30) should receive anticoagulation and evaluation for surgical thromboembolectomy. Patients with PAH should also receive **anticoagulation** to prevent microthrombi or the devastating effect of an acute thromboembolus (Chapter 30). Diuretics are used to reduce peripheral oedema.

Management of PAH is limited to treatment of symptoms and slowing progression; there is no cure. Type 5 phosphodiesterase inhibitors (e.g. sildenafil) increase cGMP and consequently augment vasorelaxation and reduce vascular remodelling; they effectively reduce symptoms (SUPER-1 study), and they are a mainstay of treatment. Endothelin-receptor antagonists (e.g. bosentan, dual ET_A and ET_B antagonist) block the action of endothelin-1, a potent vasoconstrictor and inducer of proliferation implicated in the pathogenesis of PAH. Trials (BREATHE-1, ARIES-1,-2) have shown that these drugs improve function, symptoms and exercise capacity in PAH. Chronic infusion or inhalation of stable **prostacyclin** analogues (which increase cAMP) are the only therapy shown to prolongs survival; they cause vasodilatation, inhibit vascular remodelling and may improve endothelial function. A minority of patients respond to calcium channel blockers. Lung transplantation is reserved for failed medical therapy.

30 Venous thromboembolism and pulmonary embolism

Figure 30a Pulmonary angiograms (A, D) and V/Q scans (B, E = ventilation scans, C, F = perfusion scans) in a healthy patient and a patient with a massive right-sided pulmonary embolism. The angiogram (D) shows complete occlusion of the right pulmonary artery. On the V/Q scan there is loss of right lung perfusion (F) but normal ventilation (E)

Normal

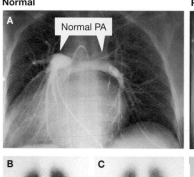

Pulmonary embolism

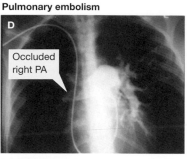

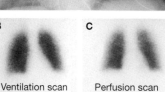

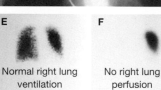

Figure 30b Contrast CT scan showing contrast in the heart and pulmonary arteries (PA). Both the right and left PA show irregular defects, consistent with pulmonary emboli

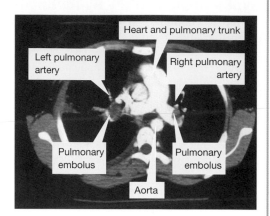

Figure 30c Risk factors for DVT and PE

Surgery	Hip, knee, gynaecological procedures
Trauma	Spinal trauma
General factors	Age, obesity, smoking, oral contraceptive pill (OCP)
Underlying disease	Malignancy, sepsis, stroke, autoimmune disease
Cardiovascular disease	Low flow states (e.g. cardiac failure and immobility) Vascular injury (e.g. atherosclerosis and catheters)
Inherited disorders (less common)	Deficiencies (e.g. antithrombin III, protein C and protein S) Clotting disorders (e.g. factor V leiden, antiphospholipid syndrome and dysfibrinogenaemias)

Figure 30d DVT prophylaxis

Risk of DVT	Patient	Regime
Low (<1%)	<40 years old, minor surgery (<1 h) Minimal immobility	Early ambulation Compression stockings
Moderate (5–10%)	>40 years old, surgery (>1 h), cardiac, medical problems, CVA, hypercoagulability	Low-dose heparin (UFH or LMWH)
High (>15%)	Complicated surgery, hip or knee surgery, hip fracture, trauma	Full-dose LMWH or warfarin

Note: the Factor X antagonist rivaroxaban is now recommended by NICE as a possible prophylactic treatment for adults with PE or DVT

LMWH = low-molecular-weight heparin
UFH = unfractionated heparin
CVA = cerebrovascular accident

The Respiratory System at a Glance, Fourth Edition. Jeremy P.T. Ward. © Jeremy P.T. Ward. Published 2015 by John Wiley & Sons, Ltd.

Venous thromboembolism and its most significant complication, **pulmonary embolism (PE)**, are common clinical disorders that have a substantial impact on patient morbidity and mortality; Figure 30c shows major risks. PE is most often a complication of **deep venous thrombosis (DVT)**. Both disorders are commonly underdiagnosed and require appropriate clinical suspicion and a systematic diagnostic approach. About 5 million patients develop DVT in the USA each year; approximately 500,000 subsequently develop PE and approximately 10% of these die. Prophylactic therapy in patients at risk is essential (Fig. 30d); in its absence up to 70% of patients undergoing hip or knee replacement surgery develop DVT.

Deep venous thrombosis

Nearly all clinically significant cases of PE (~90%) arise from DVT in the lower extremities, with thrombi typically originating in the calves and propagating above the knee. Approximately 15–25% will propagate into the femoral and iliac veins and have a 50% risk of embolizing to the lung. Thrombi may develop in the axillary and subclavian veins, usually due to surgery or intravenous catheters, but emboli are usually smaller, with less risk of catastrophic consequences. Soon after thrombus formation, the intrinsic fibrinolytic cascade begins to organize the thrombus. The risk of a thrombus embolizing is greatest early during ongoing proliferation and decreases once it is organized.

Pulmonary embolism

When a thrombus embolizes to the lung, respiratory or circulatory abnormalities occur due to sudden occlusion of a pulmonary artery or arteriole. Occlusion of regional perfusion causes an increase in dead space, necessitating an **increase in minute ventilation** to maintain normal $P_a\text{CO}_2$. Surfactant production distal to the embolus may be reduced after 24 hours, resulting in **atelectasis**. **Hypoxaemia** is common and mostly due to V_A/Q mismatch (Chapter 15). **Pulmonary infarction** occurs in less than 25% of cases of PE. Circulatory complications arise from obliteration of the pulmonary vascular bed and a reduction of cardiac output. Severity is related to the amount of lung embolized and the pre-existing state of the pulmonary vasculature and right ventricle (RV). A single large embolus can be catastrophic, whereas multiple small emboli can cause 'pruning' of smaller arteries. Circulatory collapse may occur with more than 50% obstruction of the pulmonary vascular bed. Less severe emboli may be fatal to patients with pre-existing lung or heart disease.

Clinical features

Clinical features of DVT are non-specific, with lower extremity pain, swelling and erythema. Homan's sign (pain in the calf on dorsiflexion of the foot) occurs in a minority of patients. Fifty per cent of DVTs are undetected.

Most patients with PE have **dyspnoea**, **pleuritic chest pain**, **haemoptysis**, **apprehension** and **tachypnoea**. With severe PE, signs related to **RV failure** (e.g. hypotension and jugular venous distension) may occur. Most patients with PE have non-specific abnormalities on chest X-ray, including atelectasis. The electrocardiogram (ECG) may show non-specific ST segment changes, and rarely, with significant RV strain, an $S_1Q_3T_3$ pattern (prominent S in lead I, Q and inverted T in lead III), right axis deviation (RAD) or right bundle–branch block (RBBB). **Arterial blood gas abnormalities** are common, including **widened A–a gradient**, **hypoxaemia** and **hypocapnia** (despite increased dead space).

Diagnosis

Deep venography or **pulmonary angiography** is the diagnostic standard, although **V/Q scanning** is usually the initial investigation as it is less invasive (Fig. 30a; Chapter 23). A negative perfusion scan effectively rules out PE and a 'high-probability' scan (multiple segmental perfusion defects with normal ventilation) has a more than 85% probability of PE (Fig. 30a). With a high clinical suspicion, a high-probability V/Q scan has a positive predictive value of more than 95%. Unfortunately, most V/Q scans are non-diagnostic or indeterminate, with a 15–50% likelihood of PE, necessitating further imaging. **Non-invasive imaging** of the lower extremity deep veins with Doppler imaging or impedance plethysmography is useful, because the presence of thrombosis requires treatment similar to PE. In patients with underlying cardiac or pulmonary disease, **pulmonary angiography** is indicated if the above tests are non-diagnostic. Absence of DVT and a low-probability V/Q scan permit treatment to be withheld. **Spiral/helical computed tomography** (CT) has a sensitivity for PE of 70–95% (higher for more proximal emboli) and a specificity of more than 90%. It also allows visualization of parenchymal abnormalities and is used in patients with chronic obstructive pulmonary disease (COPD) or extensive chest X-ray abnormalities, where V/Q scanning is indeterminate. **Echocardiography** may reveal RV dysfunction in PE and rule out **pericardial tamponade** or severe left ventricular (LV) dysfunction. **Transoesophageal echocardiography** may visualize thromboemboli in the main pulmonary arteries, but not in lobar or segmental arteries.

Treatment

The cornerstone of therapy for DVT/PE is **anticoagulation**, which stops propagation of existing thrombus and allows organization. Immediate therapy in patients with a high suspicion of PE may prevent further life-threatening embolization. Standard therapy is **unfractionated heparin (UFH)** or **low-molecular-weight heparin (LMWH)** for 5–7 days, followed by **warfarin** for 3–6 months. UFH and warfarin must be monitored as subtherapeutic levels increase the risk of recurrent thromboembolism. LMWH is more bioavailable and does not require monitoring. The direct Factor X antagonist rivaroxaban is now recommended by NICE as a possible alternative treatment for adults with PE and for DVT/PE prophylaxis. Patients with inherited or acquired hypercoagulability may require lifelong therapy.

In patients with contraindications to anticoagulation (recent surgery, haemorrhagic stroke, central nervous system metastases, active bleeding) or recurrent PE while on therapeutic anticoagulation, an **inferior vena cava (IVC) filter** may prevent fatal PE.

Although activation of **fibrinolysis** with **thrombolytics** hastens resolution of perfusion defects and RV dysfunction, convincing benefit is lacking. As thrombolytics cause increased bleeding complications, including a 0.3–1.5% risk of intracerebral haemorrhage, they are only recommended for life-threatening PE with compromised haemodynamics.

31 Pulmonary vasculitis

Figure 31a CT scan of patient with Wegener's granulomatosis, showing large cavitating masses

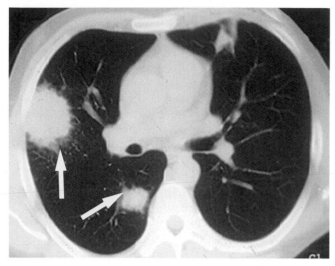

Figure 31b Histological section showing necrobiotic regions with multinucleate giant cells (arrows)

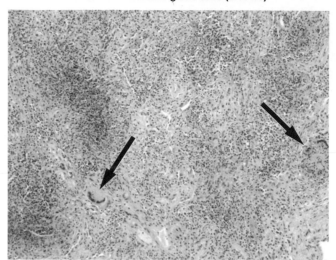

Table 1 Types and features of vasculitis

Disease	Feature	Diagnostic antibodies	Comment
Collagen vascular disease			
Rheumatoid arthritis	Arteries		Uncommon
Scleroderma	Fibrosis in arterioles		CREST syndrome
SLE	Capillaritis		Alveolar haemorrhage
Vasculitides			
Wegener's granulomatosis	Granulomatous inflammation Arteriolar/venular vasculitis Capillaritis, fibrinoid necrosis	PR3-ANCA >> MPO-ANCA	Alveolar haemorrhage
Churg–Strauss syndrome	Necrotizing vasculitis in small arteries, arterioles and venules Granulomas, eosinophils Fibrinoid necrosis	MPO-ANCA >> PR3-ANCA	Asthma, eosinophilia
Microscopic polyangiitis	Arteriole/venule vasculitis Capillaritis, fibrinoid necrosis	MPO-ANCA > PRS-ANCA	Related to Wegener's Hepatitis B, C
Goodpasture's syndrome	Intra-alveolar haemorrhage Linear IgG in basement membrane Minimal inflammation	Anti-GBM antibodies Occassionally PR3-ANCA	Alveolar haemorrhage Smoking, recent infection
Lymphomatoid granulomatosis	Angiodestructive lymphocytes Plasma cells, atypical lymphocytes		Epstein–Barr virus Lymphoproliferative

The Respiratory System at a Glance, Fourth Edition. Jeremy P.T. Ward. © Jeremy P.T. Ward. Published 2015 by John Wiley & Sons, Ltd.

Vasculitis is primarily associated with inflammation and necrosis of blood vessels, and includes a number of rare conditions (**vasculitides**) with high untreated mortality. Pulmonary vasculitis commonly occurs with systemic vasculitis, and may cause wheeze, hypoxaemia, pulmonary infiltrates, masses, necrotizing lesions and/or alveolar haemorrhage. Vasculitis may be secondary to systemic **collagen vascular disease** – such as **rheumatoid arthritis**, **scleroderma** or **systemic lupus erythematosus (SLE)** – or may be **primary vasculitides** that involve pulmonary blood vessels (**Wegener's granulomatosis (WG)**, **Churg–Strauss syndrome, microscopic polyangiitis, lymphomatoid granulomatosis** and **angiitis**). Anti-glomerular basement membrane disease (anti-GBM; **Goodpasture's syndrome**) has a similar clinical presentation to pulmonary vasculitis.

Most primary vasculitides involve neutrophil infiltration into the lung interstitium, with consequent vascular damage by fibrinoid necrosis; capillary rupture can lead to alveolar haemorrhage. Autoantibodies against components of the cytoplasm of granulocytes and neutrophils, **anti-neutrophil cytoplasmic antibodies (ANCA)**, are diagnostic markers for vasculitis and may be part of the pathology. These are differentially characterized by neutrophil staining: cytoplasmic (c-ANCA) and perinuclear (p-ANCA), which are largely synonymous with PR3-ANCA (targeting peroxidase-3), and MPO-ANCA (targeting myeloperoxidase), respectively (Table 1).

Collagen vascular diseases

Rheumatoid arthritis may cause vasculitis and **pulmonary hypertension** (Chapter 29); however, this is far less frequent than pleural disease (Chapter 34) or diffuse parenchymal disease (Chapter 32). Patients may develop **Caplan's syndrome** as a result of dust inhalation (e.g. coal dust) (Chapter 35). **Limited cutaneous scleroderma** often spares lung parenchyma and causes pulmonary hypertension by direct involvement of pulmonary arterioles. While not common, **pulmonary capillaritis** causing alveolar haemorrhage secondary to **SLE** is a devastating complication with a high mortality rate. Patients generally have a pre-existing diagnosis of SLE, usually with renal involvement. Rarely, SLE may cause pulmonary hypertension by direct involvement of the pulmonary vasculature. Clinically, this is indistinguishable from **pulmonary arterial hypertension** (Chapter 29).

Vasculitides

WG is a systemic vasculitis that predominantly involves the upper and lower respiratory systems and the renal glomeruli. Vascular inflammation may involve arterioles, capillaries and venules. Patients are generally aged 40–60 years and present with upper respiratory symptoms, usually involving the sinuses (sinusitis) or nasopharynx (ulcers, septal perforation, saddle nose deformity). Radiographic abnormalities in the chest are common, mostly as nodules or masses, often with cavitation (Fig. 31a), but they may appear as parenchymal infiltrates. Renal disease is usual and consists of glomerulonephritis with haematuria, proteinuria and red blood cell casts. Necrotizing **granulomas** (chronically inflamed tissue masses characterized by multinucleate giant cells) are seen in the lungs (Fig. 31b), nasopharynx and kidneys. WG may also involve the ears (otitis media), eyes (conjunctivitis, uveitis), heart (coronary arteries), peripheral nervous system, skin or joints. PR3-ANCA has a 60–90% sensitivity and more than 90% specificity for WG.

Churg–Strauss syndrome (*allergic granulomatosis* and *angiitis*) is a medium/small vessel granulomatous vasculitis of the lung, skin, heart, nervous system and kidney. It is probably the second most common pulmonary vasculitis after WG. Most patients have a history of allergic rhinitis and/or asthma and peripheral eosinophilia that may predate the vasculitis by up to a decade. Patients will present with worsening asthma, fever, malaise, subcutaneous tender nodules, mononeuritis multiplex and radiographic infiltrates. There may also be pericarditis, abdominal pain and glomerulonephritis. Radiographic abnormalities are most often patchy, fleeting infiltrates, but may include cavitating nodules or masses, interstitial infiltrates or pleural effusions. CT scans may show ground glass opacities or peribronchial thickening. Lung biopsy shows perivascular granulomatous inflammation, small artery and vein vasculitis, prominent eosinophils and necrosis. The diagnosis may be made without biopsy in the presence of asthma, eosinophilia, migratory pulmonary infiltrates and neuropathy. Both PR3-ANCA and MPO-ANCA may be positive. **Treatment:** most patients respond to corticosteroids. Cyclophosphamide or azathioprine may be added in resistant cases (suppress immune system). Patients who respond to therapy seldom relapse. Patients with an onset of asthma immediately before or concurrent with vasculitis have a poorer prognosis. Overall, survival is more than 70%, with increased mortality due to cardiac, central nervous system (CNS), renal or gastrointestinal involvement.

Microscopic polyangiitis has microscopic similarities to WG and polyarteritis nodosa. In contrast to WG, MPA does not involve the nasopharynx and sinuses and is usually associated with MPO-ANCA rather than PR3-ANCA. It is often seen in patients with hepatitis B or C infection. **Treatment** with corticosteroids and cyclophosphamide substantially reduces mortality.

Goodpasture's syndrome is a facet of **anti-GBM** disease, when antibodies (linear IgG) are deposited on the basement membranes of the alveoli and glomerulus, causing damage to collagen and consequent alveolar haemorrhage and glomerulonephritis, respectively. Alveolar haemorrhage occurs predominantly in smokers, or after recent respiratory infections that alter alveolar permeability. Patients present with rapidly progressive glomerulonephritis, haemoptysis, anaemia and diffuse alveolar infiltrates on radiographs. In contrast to the primary vasculitides, prolonged systemic symptoms are uncommon. Pulmonary function testing demonstrates elevated $D_L$co from extravasated haemoglobin in the lung. Diagnosis requires demonstration of anti-GBM antibodies in serum or linear IgG in glomerular or alveolar basement membranes. Both PR3-ANCA and MPO-ANCA may be positive. **Treatment:** patients with Goodpasture's syndrome should be treated with high-dose corticosteroids, cyclophosphamide and sometimes plasmapheresis. Therapy may control alveolar haemorrhage, but pulmonary and renal function may not recover.

Lymphomatoid granulomatosis is a systemic vasculitis of lungs, kidneys, CNS and skin. It is strongly associated with, and may be a late complication of, **Epstein–Barr virus** infection. It behaves like an indolent lymphoproliferative disease and may transform into a B-cell lymphoma. Patients typically have fever, malaise, cough, dyspnoea and a papular rash. Radiographic abnormalities usually consist of multiple lower lobe nodular densities. Lung biopsy shows angiocentric/angiodestructive mixed cell infiltration with lymphocytes, plasma cells and atypical lymphocytes. Vascular occlusion and necrosis are common. **Treatment:** Lymphomatoid granulomatosis is considered to be a lymphoproliferative disorder and is treated with chemotherapy and corticosteroids. Without treatment, the disease progresses and is usually fatal.

32 Diffuse parenchymal (interstitial) lung diseases

Figure 32a   Classification ▇ and diagnostic ▇ process in DPLD

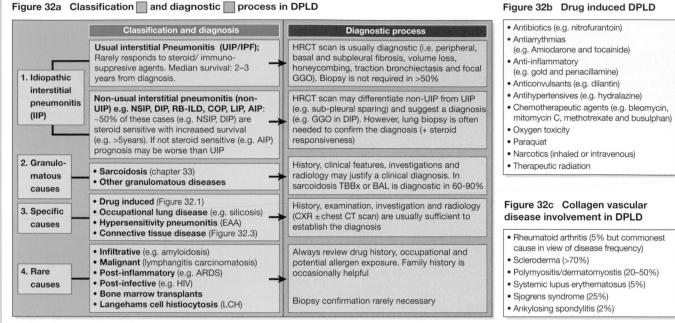

Classification and diagnosis		Diagnostic process
1. Idiopathic interstitial pneumonitis (IIP)	**Usual interstitial Pneumonitis (UIP/IPF);** Rarely responds to steroid/ immuno-suppresive agents. Median survival: 2–3 years from diagnosis.	HRCT scan is usually diagnostic (i.e. peripheral, basal and subpleural fibrosis, volume loss, honeycombing, traction bronchiectasis and focal GGO). Biopsy is not required in >50%
	Non-usual interstitial pneumonitis (non-UIP) e.g. NSIP, DIP, RB-ILD, COP, LIP, AIP: ~50% of these cases (e.g. NSIP, DIP) are steroid sensitive with increased survival (e.g. >5years). If not steroid sensitive (e.g. AIP) prognosis may be worse than UIP	HRCT scan may differentiate non-UIP from UIP (e.g. sub-pleural sparing) and suggest a diagnosis (e.g. GGO in DIP). However, lung biopsy is often needed to confirm the diagnosis (+ steroid responsiveness)
2. Granulo-matous causes	• Sarcoidosis (chapter 33) • Other granulomatous diseases	History, clinical features, investigations and radiology may justify a clinical diagnosis. In sarcoidosis TBBx or BAL is diagnostic in 60-90%
3. Specific causes	• Drug induced (Figure 32.1) • Occupational lung disease (e.g. silicosis) • Hypersensitivity pneumonitis (EAA) • Connective tissue disease (Figure 32.3)	History, examination, investigation and radiology (CXR ± chest CT scan) are usually sufficient to establish the diagnosis
4. Rare causes	• Infiltrative (e.g. amyloidosis) • Malignant (lymphangitis carcinomatosis) • Post-inflammatory (e.g. ARDS) • Post-infective (e.g. HIV) • Bone marrow transplants • Langehams cell histiocytosis (LCH)	Always review drug history, occupational and potential allergen exposure. Family history is occasionally helpful Biopsy confirmation rarely necessary

Figure 32b   Drug induced DPLD

- Antibiotics (e.g. nitrofurantoin)
- Antiarrythmias (e.g. Amiodarone and tocainide)
- Anti-inflammatory (e.g. gold and penacillamine)
- Anticonvulsants (e.g. dilantin)
- Antihypertensives (e.g. hydralazine)
- Chemotherapeutic agents (e.g. bleomycin, mitomycin C, methotrexate and busulphan)
- Oxygen toxicity
- Paraquat
- Narcotics (inhaled or intravenous)
- Therapeutic radiation

Figure 32c   Collagen vascular disease involvement in DPLD

- Rheumatoid arthritis (5% but commonest cause in view of disease frequency)
- Scleroderma (>70%)
- Polymyositis/dermatomyostis (20–50%)
- Systemic lupus erythematosus (5%)
- Sjogrens syndrome (25%)
- Ankylosing spondylitis (2%)

IPF = idiopathic pulmonary fibrosis; TBBx = transbronchial biopsy; BAL = bronchioalveolar lavage; UIP = usual interstitial pneumonia; NSIP = non-specific interstitial pneumonia; DIP = desquamative interstitial pneumonia; RB = respiratory bronchiolitis; AIP = acute interstitial pneumonia; COP= organising pneumonia; LIP = lymphoctic interstitial pneumonia; DPLD=diffuse parenchymal lung disease; CTD=connective tissue disease ARDS =acute respiratory distress syndrome; EAA = extrinsic allergic allveolitis); HRCT= High resolution CT scan; GGO = ground glass opacification

Figure 32d   HRCT scan showing subpleural honeycomb fibrosis in UIP

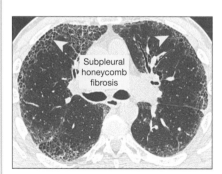

Figure 32e   HRCT scan showing subpleural sparing, coarse reticular shadowing and traction bronchiectasis in NSIP

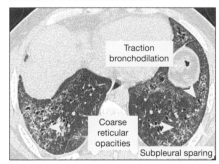

Figure 32f   HRCT scan showing ground glass opacification (GGO) and mosaic pattern typical of alveolitis in DIP

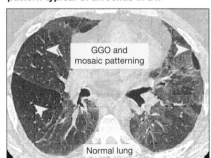

Figure 32g   Clinical features, age at onset, histologic pattern and radiographic features of idiopathic interstitial pneumonias

Clinical name	Age, sex	Clinical features, relation to smoking and response to treatment	Typical CT findings
UIP/IPF	50–80 yrs M>>F	Gradual onset. Acute exacerbations. Worse in smokers. BAL shows neutrophils (±eosinophils). Poor response to steroids and immunosuppressive agents. Median survival 2–3 years from diagnosis	Subpleural, peripheral and mainly basal reticulation, volume loss, honeycombing, traction bronchiectasis and focal GGO
NSIP	40–50 yrs M=F	Gradual onset 6–30 months or subacute. Not related to smoking. BAL lymphocytosis. Prognosis better than UIP, especially in cellular (inflammatory) disease. Most patients improve or recover with steroid (±immunosuppressive) therapy	Peripheral and mainly basal GGO, consolidation and reticular opacities with subpleural sparing
DIP	40–50 yrs M>>F	A form of severe RB-ILD. Characterized by BAL pigment-laden alveolar macrophages which fill alveolar spaces. Nearly always due to smoking. Prognosis >10 years following smoking cessation and/or steroid therapy in 70%. Progression to fibrosis in <20%.	Mainly lower zone and peripheral. GGO++ and reticular lines. Mosaic pattern of normal and abnormal lung
AIP	Any age M=F	Rapidly progressive disease, indistinguishable from ARDS. Often presents after a viral URTI. No effective therapy and mortality is >50% and occurs within 4–8 weeks of onset. Recurrence or progressive fibrosis may occur in survivors.	Widespread, diffuse consolidation and GGO (lobular sparing). Late traction bronchiectasis

IPF = idiopathic pulmonary fibrosis; UIP = usual interstitial pneumonia; NSIP = non-specific interstitial pneumonia; DIP = desquamative interstitial pneumonia; RB = respiratory bronchiolitis; RB-ILD = respiratory bronchiolitis-interstitial lung disease; AIP = acute interstitial pneumonia; DAD = diffuse alveolar damage; COP = cryptogenic organizing pneumonia; LIP = lymphocytic interstitial pneumonia; GGO = ground glass opacification; BAL = bronchoalveolar lavage; CTD = connective tissue disease, SLE = systemic lupus erythematosus

Diffuse parenchymal (interstitial) lung diseases (DPLD/ILD) are characterized by inflammation and/or fibrosis of the pulmonary interstitium (i.e. tissue between the alveolar epithelium and capillary endothelium) and the bronchovascular and septal tissues comprising the lung's fibrous framework. The alveolar airspaces, distal airways and vasculature may also be involved.

Clinical features

Insidious onset of dyspnoea, cough, bilateral inspiratory crackles (±finger clubbing) and exercise-induced desaturation are common to all DPLD. Hypoxaemia and right heart failure occur in advanced disease. *Pulmonary function tests* (PFT) reveal a restrictive defect with reduced total lung capacity (TLC), functional residual capacity (FRC) and residual volume (RV) due to impaired lung compliance. Gas transfer (DL_{CO}) decreases due to diminished surface area for gas exchange. *Chest X-ray* (CXR) abnormalities (>90%) include mainly lower lobe alveolar, interstitial or mixed infiltrates. *Bronchoalveolar lavage* (BAL) excludes other diseases (e.g. malignancy). An increase in BAL inflammatory cells indicates alveolitis and correlates with ground glass opacification (GGO) on high resolution computed tomography (HRCT) scans and reflects rapidly progressive or potentially reversible disease. *HRCT scans (±histology)* are required for classification.

Classification

There are four main categories of DPLD (Fig. 32a) with considerable overlap.

1 **Idiopathic interstitial pneumonitis** (IIP) comprises two distinct subgroups.
- *Usual Interstitial pneumonia* (UIP; previously known as idiopathic pulmonary fibrosis (IPF) or cryptogenic fibrosing alveolitis), causes ~70% of IIP. *Pathogenesis:* there is minimal inflammation in UIP. Fibroblast proliferation with abnormal alveolar epithelial healing causes fibrosis. *Incidence* is ~$5/10^5$/year and it affects older men, aged ~70 years old. *Clinical features* include progressive dyspnoea interspersed with acute 'exacerbations', cough, clubbing (~25–50%) and basal inspiratory crepitations. *HRCT scans* show bilateral, basal, subpleural reticular changes with honeycombing and traction bronchiectasis (Fig. 32d). Consolidation, GGO and nodules are infrequent. *Histology* reveals peripheral, patchy fibrosis and honeycombing alternating with areas of normal lung, similar to that in asbestosis, collagen vascular and drug-induced DPLD. Diffuse alveolar damage (DAD) and cryptogenic organising pneumonia (COP) occur during acute exacerbations. *Treatment:* UIP does not respond to steroids or immunosuppressants. *Median survival* from diagnosis is <3 years and worse in smokers.
- *Non-usual interstitial pneumonitis* (non-UIP) causes ~30% of IIP. Differences in clinical course, histology, HRCT and outcome suggest that these rare disorders are distinct clinicopathologic entities (Fig. 32g). They include (in order of frequency), non-specific interstitial pneumonitis (NSIP), COP previously known as bronchiolitis obliterans organizing pneumonia (BOOP), acute interstitial pneumonia (AIP; formerly known as Hamman–Rich syndrome), respiratory bronchiolitis-interstitial lung disease (RB-ILD), desquamative interstitial pneumonitis (DIP) and lymphoid interstitial pneumonitis (LIP). Presentation is earlier than UIP, mainly in men, aged 40–50 years old. Pulmonary involvement is more diffuse, more cellular and less fibrotic with subpleural sparing (Fig. 32e), than UIP. HRCT scans often show bilateral, widespread, subpleural or basal GGO (Fig. 32f). Non-UIP is sensitive to steroid (±immunosuppressive) therapy, with a median survival >10 years, in 50% of cases. In steroid-resistant disease (e.g. AIP) prognosis may be worse than in UIP (e.g. <6 months).

2 DPLD due to specific causes; includes
- *Drug-induced DPLD* (Fig. 32b). Mechanisms include oxidant-mediated injury (e.g. nitrofurantoin), direct cytotoxic effects (e.g. bleomycin), cellular phospholipid deposition (e.g. amiodarone) and immune-mediated injury (e.g. hydralazine). Treatment includes drug withdrawal and occasionally steroid therapy. Irreversible damage causes respiratory failure (e.g. amiodarone).
- *Hypersensitivity pneumonitis* (HP; also known as extrinsic allergic alveolitis) is discussed in Chapter 35. It is an inflammatory response to inhaled, mainly organic antigens, to which the patient has become sensitised (e.g. thermophilic actinomycetes from mouldy hay in farmer's lung).
- *Connective tissue disease (CTD) DPLD* occurs in 5% of rheumatoid arthritis (RA) patients, especially those with multisystem disease (e.g. vasculitis) but is usually asymptomatic. Symptomatic ILD occurs in other CTD (Fig. 32c) and after some treatments (e.g. methotrexate). NSIP is the usual histological pattern except in RA, where 50% have a UIP pattern.
- *Occupational lung disease* follows inhalation of mainly mineral (e.g. coal, asbestos) dusts (Chapter 35).

3 **Granulomatous DPLD:** sarcoidosis, the second most frequent DPLD and other granulomatous DPLD are discussed in Chapter 33.

4 **Rare causes of DPLD:** include infiltrative, malignant and post inflammatory/infective causes, bone marrow transplantation and rare lung diseases (e.g. Langerhans cell histiocytosis).

Diagnosis

Diagnosis of DPLD due to occupational exposure, drugs, CTD, HP or sarcoidosis often follows a comprehensive history, careful examination, blood tests, serology (e.g. avian precipitans), PFT and radiological imaging (Fig. 32a). In contrast, initial diagnosis of IIP is one of exclusion. Subsequent classification, to distinguish UIP from other IIP (e.g. NSIP), has important therapeutic and prognostic implications and requires an integrated clinical, radiological and pathological approach. *HRCT scans* aid this differentiation. Typical clinical and HRCT features allow confident diagnosis of UIP and avoids the need for biopsy in ~50% of cases. *Surgical biopsy* is considered if radiology is not diagnostic and in non-UIP. Transbronchial biopsies are inadequate for histological classification but may be diagnostic in sarcoidosis.

Management

Treatment is considered in patients with deteriorating symptoms, inflammatory changes (e.g. GGO) or if requested despite poor evidence for benefit (e.g. UIP). *Supportive therapy* requires supplemental oxygen, pulmonary rehabilitation, nutrition, smoking cessation and palliative care. *Pharmacological therapy* includes steroids and/or immunosuppressive agents (e.g. azathioprine, methotrexate). In steroid sensitive conditions (e.g. DIP, NSIP) a short trial of high dose steroids may be indicated. In patients requiring ongoing therapy or those less likely to respond (e.g. UIP), combination therapy with low dose prednisolone, azathioprine and N-acetylcysteine is sometimes recommended. In many patients, therapy is ineffective and has significant side effects. Consider referral for lung transplantation.

33 Sarcoidosis

Figure 33a Causes of lung granuloma

Idiopathic: Sarcoidosis

Infective: Tuberculosis, leprosy, brucellosis, fungal, schistosomiasis, cat-scratch fever, syphilis

Malignancy: Lymphoma

Gastrointestinal: Crohn's disease, primary biliary cirrhosis

Allergic: Extrinsic allergic alveolitis

Occupational: Berylliosis, silicosis

Vasculitic: Wegener's granulomatosis, giant cell arteritis, polyarteritis nodosa, Takyasu's arteritis

Others: Thyroiditis, Langerhans' cell histiocytosis, hypogammaglobulinaemia, orchitis

Figure 33c Initial evaluation of sarcoidosis

History (+occupational/environmental exposure)

Examination including fundoscopy

Full blood count, biochemistry, calcium, liver function, LDH, SACE

ECG, CXR, Urine analysis (±calcium excretion)

Spirometry and gas transfer (DLCO)

Mantoux test (to exclude tuberculosis)

LDH = lacate dehydrogenase; SACE = serum angiotensin-converting enzyme; ECG = electrocardiogram; CXR = chest X-ray

Figure 33b Characteristic CXR features in pulmonary sarcoidosis

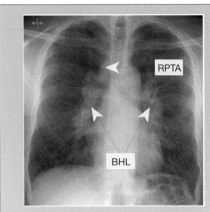

(i) **Bilhilar lymphadenopathy (BHL) and right paratracheal adenopathy (RPTA)**

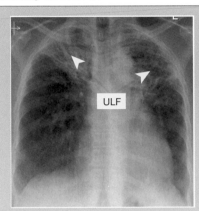

(ii) **Upper lobe fibrosis (ULF)**

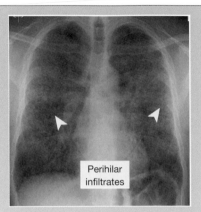

(iii) **Perihilar infiltrates**

Figure 33d Radiographic staging in sarcoidosis and likelihood of spontaneous resolution

Stage	Finding	Likelihood of spontaneous resolution
0	Normal chest radiograph	>90%
I	Bilateral hilar lymphadenopathy (BHL)	60–90%
II	BHL plus pulmonary infiltrates	40–60%
III	Pulmonary infiltrates (without BHL)	10–20%
IV	Pulmonary fibrosis (± bullae)	<20%

Figure 33e CT scan of pulmonary sarcoidosis showing hilar adenopathy and peri-bronchovascular nodules. Inset shows fissural nodules/'beading' on HRCT

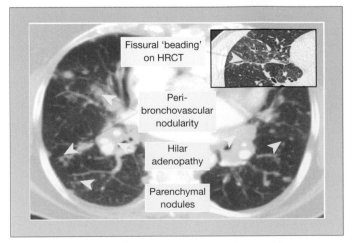

Figure 33f Criteria for steroid therapy in sarcoidosis

Progressive symptomatic pulmonary disease

Asymptomatic pulmonary disease with ongoing loss of lung function

Cardiac disease

Neurological disease

Eye disease not responding to topical therapy

Symptomatic hypercalcaemia

Other symptomatic/progressive extrapulmonary disease

Sarcoidosis is a multisystem disorder and although predominantly respiratory (>90%), many tissues can be affected. It usually presents in 20–40 year olds, most frequently the Irish, Afro-Caribbeans, Scandinavians and relatives of sarcoid patients. Black people are more susceptible to aggressive, systemic disease. *Incidence* varies geographically from 5–100/10^5/population.

Aetiology is unknown but it often occurs in a genetically susceptible person (e.g. HLA-DR) exposed to an antigenic trigger which may be infective (e.g. mycobacteria, propionibacteria), geographical (e.g. pine pollen) or occupational (e.g. beryllium). Autoimmune causes are less likely. **Histopathology** is characterized by non-caseating granulomata (NCG) and an abnormal, antigen-triggered CD4 (helper) T-cell response. Interferon gamma production stimulates granuloma formation, fibroblasts and fibrosis and activated macrophages release serum angiotensin converting enzyme (SACE). Delayed hypersensitivity (e.g. to tuberculin) is reduced. Figure 33a illustrates other causes of lung granuloma.

Clinical features are pulmonary (>90%), systemic or both.

1 Pulmonary sarcoidosis may be asymptomatic (~30%) or associated with constitutional (e.g. fever, malaise, weight loss ~30%; fatigue ~70%) and/or respiratory (e.g. dry cough, dyspnoea ~30–50%) symptoms. Physical findings are rare (i.e. despite CXR infiltrates, crepitations occur in <20% of cases). There are two distinct pulmonary presentations:

a *Acute sarcoidosis* (Löfgren's syndrome); usually affects Caucasians with fever, erythema nodosum (EN), arthralgia bihilar lymphadenopathy (BHL; Fig. 33b.i) and/or pulmonary infiltrates which may be asymptomatic CXR findings. Exclude other causes of BHL (e.g. TB, lymphoma). Pulmonary fibrosis develops in ~10%.

b *Progressive, interstitial lung disease* with dyspnoea and cough which may progress to pulmonary fibrosis and respiratory failure. CXR (Figs. 33b.ii, 33b.iii) reveals fibrosis and/or infiltrates (±BHL).

Diagnosis depends on clinical (±CXR) features; histological detection of NCG and exclusion of other causes (e.g. TB). Figure 33c summarizes initial evaluation. *Disease progression* is monitored by serial clinical assessment, CXR, spirometry (±DLCO) and SACE.

• *SACE* increases in 80% of acute sarcoidosis and falls with steroid therapy. Although non-specific (i.e. raised in TB) it aids monitoring.

• *CXR* is abnormal in >85% of cases (Fig. 33b) but 30–60% are asymptomatic (i.e. incidental CXR finding). BHL occurs in 50–85%, unilateral hilar lymphadenopathy in <10% and central or upper lobe pulmonary infiltrates in 25–50% of cases. Figure 33d shows the CXR staging system.

• *High resolution CT scans* are not required for routine evaluation but if the CXR is normal, may discriminate between inflammation and fibrosis and detect complications. Characteristic features include bronchovascular micronodules (Fig. 33e), inflammation with ground glass opacification and septal thickening. Later disease causes traction bronchiectasis and fibrosis.

• *Histological confirmation* is not needed in asymptomatic or acute disease. It is recommended in symptomatic cases or if BHL is asymmetrical or massive (to exclude malignancy; ~10%). Histological diagnosis is usually obtained from transbronchial lung (~70%) or occasionally tissue (e.g. parotid) biopsies. A positive Mantoux test makes sarcoidosis unlikely.

• *Pulmonary function tests* (PFT) are abnormal in 20% of stage 1 and 40–70% of stage 2–4 radiographic disease (Fig. 33d). Restrictive PFT are typical but may be obstructive in up to 40%. Gas transfer (D_LCO) and FVC are reduced despite a normal CXR in 15–50% of cases.

Management. Most pulmonary sarcoidosis resolves spontaneously and treatment is not required (Fig. 33d). Monitor asymptomatic BHL and CXR infiltrates (stages II, III).

• *Steroid therapy* alleviates acute symptoms but does not prevent progressive pulmonary fibrosis. Figure 33f summarizes indications for treatment. Optimal dose and duration of therapy is unknown. The response to high-dose steroids is evaluated after 1–2 months. The dose is then tapered over 6–24 months. Relapse is common (>33%) and managed with prolonged low-dose steroid therapy. Prophylaxis for osteoporosis and peptic ulcers is required. The role of inhaled steroids is limited.

• *Immunosuppressive therapy* is indicated for steroid insensitive disease and as a steroid sparing agent. Methotrexate and azathioprine are beneficial in ~50% of steroid-resistant cases. Others cytotoxic agents include cyclophosphamide and cyclosporine. Hydroxychloroquine, inhibits granuloma formation and is effective for hypercalcaemia, skin, lung and neurosarcoid. Monitor toxicity.

• *Lung transplant* is considered in end-stage lung disease. NCG may recur in transplanted lung.

2 Systemic (extrathoracic) disease may cause fever, weight loss, malaise and arthralgia. Liver involvement, renal impairment (35%), splenomegaly, bone cysts and parotid, lacrimal or salivary gland swelling also occur. Hypercalcaemia, responsive to steroids, is common in men and Caucasians.

• *Skin* is often affected in women (~25%). EN describes painful, inflamed plaques usually on the shins. Lupus pernio (LP) produces indurated 'bluish', nose, ear or cheek lesions in chronic sarcoidosis. Topical steroids may be effective in EN but LP requires steroids, hydroxychloroquine (±methotrexate) therapy.

• *Eye* (e.g. uveitis, scleritis) involvement is common in women and Afro-Caribbeans. Ophthalmology assessment is essential. Treat with oral steroids (±steroid eyedrops).

• *Cardiac disease* (e.g. arrhythmias, heart failure) is uncommon (~5%) in the 'West' but causes >70% of sarcoid deaths in Japan. Treatment is with high-dose steroids, antiarrhythmics and pacemakers.

• *Neurosarcoid* (~10%) causes nerve (e.g. mononeuritis multiplex) and focal cerebral (e.g. diabetes insipidus) lesions. Steroid and immunosuppressive therapy is required.

Prognosis. Factors associated with relapse and poor outcome include age (>40 years at onset), Afro-Caribbean ethnicity, systemic disease and CXR stage (Fig. 33d). Spontaneous remission usually occurs within 3 years. Failure to remit within this time predicts a chronic course (~20%) and death in 2–5% of cases. PFT are not prognostic but serial FVC and DL_{CO} detect progressive fibrosis which causes 87% of sarcoid deaths in the USA.

34 Pleural diseases

Figure 34a   Causes of pleural effusions

Exudative	Transudative
(protein ratio pleural/serum >0.5 or LDH ratio pleural/serum >0.6 or pleural LDH >0.66 of top normal serum value)	(meets none of the criteria for exudative)

Infectious
- Para-pneumonic
  - aerobic bacterial pneumonia
  - anaerobic bacterial pneumonia
- Empyema
- Tuberculosis
- Parasitic
  - amoeba
  - echinococcus
  - paragonimus
- Viral

Autoimmune/collagen vascular
- Systemic lupus erythematosus
- Rheumatoid arthritis

Neoplastic
- Lung cancer
- Metastatic disease
- Mesothelioma

Abdominal
- Pancreatitis/pseudocyst
- Oesophageal rupture
- Liver abscess
- Splenic abscess

Miscellaneous
- Pulmonary embolism
- Drug reactions
- Asbestos exposure
- Haemothorax
- Chylothorax
- Post-cardiac surgery
- Post-myocardial infarction
- Meig's syndrome

Transudative
- Congestive heart failure
- Cirrhosis
  Hepatic hydrothorax
- Myxoedema
- Nephrotic disease
- Peritoneal dialysis

Figure 34b   CXR showing large pleural effusion in left lung (contrast with pneumothorax CXR in Chapter 37)

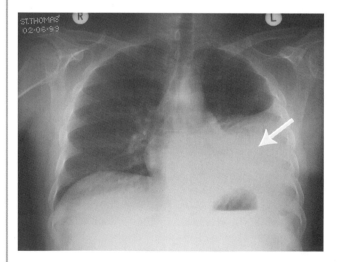

Figure 34c   CT scan demonstrating irregular (lumpy) pleural thickening of mesothelioma over lateral right chest wall (see arrows)

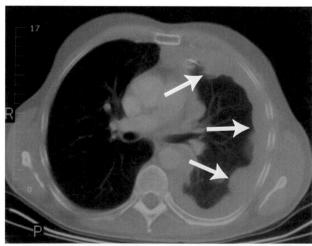

The Respiratory System at a Glance, Fourth Edition. Jeremy P.T. Ward. © Jeremy P.T. Ward. Published 2015 by John Wiley & Sons, Ltd.

The pleurae

The potential space between the **parietal** and **visceral pleurae** serves as a coupling system between the lung and the chest wall, and normally contains a small amount of fluid. A negative pleural pressure is maintained by the dynamic tension between the chest wall and the lung (Chapter 3). Both pleurae have a systemic blood supply and lymphatics, although lymphatic drainage of the pleural space is predominantly via the parietal pleura. Fluid flux through the pleural space is determined by Starling's relationship between microvascular pressures, oncotic pressures, permeability and surface area. Normally, there is net filtration of **transudative** (protein-poor) fluid into the pleural space that is balanced by resorption via the parietal lymphatics.

Pneumothorax is an important condition that occurs when air enters the pleural space and pleural pressure rises to atmospheric pressure; pneumothorax is discussed in detail in Chapter 37.

Chylothorax is due to accumulation of triglyceride-rich lymph in the pleural space, generally as the result of damage to the thoracic duct causing leakage into the pleural space, for example, due to trauma or carcinoma.

Empyema is accumulation of pus.

Pleurisy is a term commonly used to describe the sharp localized pain arising from any disease of the pleura. It is made worse by deep inspiration and coughing.

Pathophysiology

Most diseases of the pleura present with **pleural effusion**, which can be detected on chest X-ray (CXR) when more than 300 mL of fluid is present (Fig. 34b). Effusions are due to excessive fluid formation or inadequate fluid clearance. Symptoms develop if the fluid is **inflammatory** or if **pulmonary mechanics** are compromised. Thus, the most common symptoms of a pleural effusion are **pleuritic chest pain**, **dull aching pain**, **fullness of the chest** or **dyspnoea**. Physical examination reveals decreased breath sounds, dullness to percussion, decreased tactile or vocal fremitus. If there is inflammation, there may be a friction rub. **Compressive atelectasis** (partial lung collapse) may cause bronchial breath sounds.

It is useful to categorize pleural effusions as **transudative** or **exudative** (Fig. 34a).

Transudative effusions are usually due to an imbalance in Starling's forces across normal pleural membranes, have protein-poor fluid, are often bilateral and are not associated with fever, pleuritic pain or tenderness to palpation. The most common cause of a transudative effusion is **congestive heart failure**. Other causes include cirrhosis with ascites, nephrotic syndrome, pericardial disease or peritoneal dialysis.

Exudative effusions imply disease of the pleura or the adjacent lung and are characterized by an increased protein, lactate dehydrogenase (LDH), cholesterol or white blood cell count (WBC) (Fig. 34a). The differential diagnosis of exudative effusions is broad, including infection, malignancy, autoimmune disease, oesophageal perforation and pancreatitis.

Diagnostic evaluation of pleural effusion should include measurement of pleural aspirate cell count with differential, pH, protein, LDH, cholesterol and glucose. These studies usually distinguish exudates from transudates and will often suggest a specific diagnosis. For example, extremely low glucose is typical for empyema, malignancy, tuberculosis (Chapter 40), rheumatoid arthritis, systemic lupus erythematosus (SLE) or oesophageal perforation. If clinically indicated, a specific diagnosis may be obtained from microbiological stains and culture, cytopathology, amylase, triglycerides and measurement of anti-nuclear antibody (ANA) titre. Although all patients with SLE have a positive ANA titre in the pleural fluid, it is also present in a significant proportion (~15%) of other effusions; these may be related to malignancy.

Treatment is for the underlying condition, but persistent or reaccumulating effusions can be drained to dryness (slowly so as to avoid severe pain).

Specific conditions

Pneumonia (Chapters 38 and 39) commonly causes parapneumonic pleural effusions. These effusions are usually sterile exudates with a neutrophilic leukocytosis and require only treatment of the pneumonia to resolve. However, if bacteria invade the pleural space, a complicated parapneumonic effusion or empyema will develop. These effusions are characterized by a low pH and extensive fibrin deposition causing fluid loculation and require adequate open or closed drainage for healing. *Streptococcus pneumoniae*, *Staphylococcus aureus*, Gram-negative bacteria and anaerobes commonly cause complicated effusions.

Tuberculosis pleurisy occurs when a subpleural focus of primary infection ruptures into the pleural space, causing a delayed hypersensitivity response. Subsequently, an exudative effusion with a lymphocytic leukocytosis, a paucity of macrophages and an elevated adenosine deaminase will develop. Patients develop fever, dyspnoea, pleuritic pain and a positive tuberculin response (Chapter 40). Granulomatous inflammation is seen on pleural biopsy, and culture of pleural tissue has the highest diagnostic yield.

Primary lung malignancies or **metastases** to the lung may cause pleural effusions by direct invasion or by obstruction of parietal lymphatic drainage. Malignant effusions are mostly exudative (90%), often with a very high LDH, low pH and low glucose. Cytology of the pleural fluid has a high diagnostic yield. Symptomatic pleural effusions may respond to therapy for the underlying malignancy, although palliative obliteration of the pleural space (**pleurodesis**) is often necessary to relieve dyspnoea or chest pain.

Mesothelioma is an uncommon malignancy that originates in the pleura and/or peritoneum (Chapter 35). Over 75% of cases develop 20–30 years after occupational asbestos exposure. Asbestos may also cause benign pleural effusions or calcified plaques on the parietal pleura in the lower lungs or along the diaphragmatic surface. Mesothelioma typically develops in men aged 50–70 years, presenting with insidious dyspnoea and aching chest pain. CXRs usually show unilateral pleural effusion (Fig. 34b), and computed tomography (CT) shows lumpy fibrotic encasement of the pleural space (Fig. 34c). Pleural fluid cytology is not usually diagnostic. Thoracoscopic biopsies have the highest yield. Treatment is generally palliative, including pleurodesis. The prognosis is poor, with a median survival of approximately 1 year.

35 Occupational and environmental-related lung disease

Figure 35a Common examples of irritant gases and other agents causing lung-specific responses

Agent	Source	Response
Ammonia	Industrial refrigeration leaks, fertilizers	***Low exposure*** Exacerbations of asthma and COPD Enhanced response to allergen
Chlorine gas	Industrial leakage, water purification including swimming pools, household bleach (liquid/powder) interactions	***Moderate exposure*** Mild mucosal irritation Airway inflammation and bronchiolitis
Hydrogen sulphide	Sewers and manure pits, fossil fuel extraction	
Nitrogen dioxide Nitrogen oxides	Vehicle exhausts, welding, power stations, oil refineries, gas and oil burning equipment, organic decomposition, structural or polymer fires	***Severe exposure*** Epithelial damage leading to diffuse alveolar damage Pulmonary oedema and ARDS
Ozone	Vehicle exhausts, welding, copiers, ozone generators, bleaching, watertreatment, plasma welding	***In some cases – late response (2–8 weeks)*** Bronchiolitis obliterans after initial recovery
Sulphur dioxide	Combustion of fossil fuels, power stations, oil refineries, smelters, oil burning heaters, mining, ore refining, cement manufacturing, refrigeration plants	**Also:** direct bronchoconstriction, especially inasthmatics
Acrolein, aldehydes	Structural or wildland fires, other combustion	**Also:** strongly pro-inflammatory (esp. acrolein)
Diesel particulates (<10 μm)	Diesel engines	Airway/alveolar inflammationIncreased deaths in elderly
Heavy metals (cadmium, mercury)	Welding, brazing, metal cutting, metal reclamation	Acute pneumonitis 12–24 hours after exposure
Paraquat	Ingestion of herbicides	Accelerated, chemically induced pulmonary fibrosis
Polycyclic hydrocarbons Hydrocarbons	Diesel exhaust, tobacco smoke Ingestion of hydrocarbons (children)	Cancer Aspiration hydrocarbon pneumonitis

Figure 35b Typical causes of allergic alveolitis

Disease/occupation	Material	Causative agent
Farmer's lung	Mouldy hay or other vegetable matter	Thermophilic actinomycetes bacteria (*Saccharopolyspora rectivirgula*, *Thermoactinomyces* species)
Bagassosis	Sugarcane	
Mushroom workers	Compost	
Humidifier fever	Contaminated water	– Also *Klebsiella oxytoca*, amoebae
Pigeon fancier's (breeder's) lung	Feathers and excreta	Avian proteins
Farmers, sawmill, tobacco, esparto grass and brewery workers	Fungal contamination of materials	Primarily *Aspergillus* species
Cheese, laboratory, cork workers	Fungal contamination of materials	Primarily *Penicillium* species
Household	Fungal infestations of damp walls and woodwork	Multiple fungal species
– Other bacterial causes	Contamination of water, wood shavings, etc.	*Bacillus subtilis, Klebsiella, Epicoccum nigrum,* non-tubercular mycobacteria

The most common form of occupational and environmental lung disease is **asthma** (Chapters 26 and 27). The UK government has reported that 750,000 people with asthma work in an environment that triggers their symptoms, and more than 3000 per year develop asthma as a result of workplace substances. While the most common cause of occupational asthma is isocyanates (e.g. paint and plastics), grain and flour dust are not far behind, and secondary smoking is most commonly reported to exacerbate symptoms. It is estimated that elimination of occupational asthma alone could have a benefit of up to £1 billion over 10 years; education and prevention are therefore key targets. Atmospheric pollution in the form of car exhausts, diesel particulates and smoke, particularly in main roads and in cities, exacerbates symptoms of respiratory disease and can lead to increased mortality in the vulnerable and elderly.

Response to acute lung irritants

Inhaled irritants (Fig. 35a) cause exacerbation of asthma and chronic obstructive pulmonary disease (COPD), coughing and dyspnoea through activation of irritant receptors (Chapter 13), and irritation of mucous membranes. Highly soluble agents (e.g. ammonia and sulphur dioxide) cause immediate irritation in the upper airways, whereas less soluble agents (e.g. chlorine and ozone) favour deeper penetration to alveolar epithelial cells, which are particularly susceptible to injury. High concentrations lead to extensive lung injury, primarily by damage to epithelium, consequent inflammation and **pulmonary oedema**. Development of **acute respiratory distress syndrome** (ARDS) is common, and treatment is similar (Chapter 43). Some patients who initially recover from moderate or severe exposure may subsequently develop **bronchiolitis obliterans** (obliteration of bronchioles by fibrous growth) after 2–8 weeks. Although steroids may slow progression, prognosis is often poor.

Inhalation of mineral dusts (pneumoconiosis)

Coal worker's pneumoconiosis (CWP) is caused by inhalation of coal or carbon dust. In **simple CWP**, the upper lobes of the lung contain small (<4 mm), round opacities (coal macules) consisting of dust, dust-laden macrophages and fibroblasts. These may enlarge to fibrosed coal nodules. Weakening of bronchiolar walls leads to focal emphysema, which together with macules is characteristic of CWP. Simple CWP is often described as symptomless, with no change in lung function. It can however develop into **progressive massive fibrosis** (PMF), with black fibrotic masses from 1 cm to several centimetres in diameter, which may have necrotic cavities. Obliteration and disruption of airways result in emphysema. Patients show irreversible airflow limitation, loss of lung volume and elastic recoil, and reduced D_LCO, with breathlessness on exertion. Treatment is limited, and similar to other progressive fibrotic diseases (Chapter 25). **Caplan's syndrome** is a nodular form of CWP associated with the defective immunology of rheumatoid disease; it may also occur with asbestosis or silicosis.

Asbestos is a fibrous mixture of silicates that is highly resistant to degradation. The fibres are 1–2 μm wide, but up to 50 μm (**blue asbestos** – crocidolite) or 2 cm (**white asbestos** – chrysotile) long. They are thus easily trapped in the lung. Blue asbestos is far more dangerous. Regulations have reduced exposure since the 1980s, but the presence of asbestos in buildings and the long interval between exposure and disease development mean that asbestos-related disease will be encountered for some time. **Asbestos bodies** (protein-covered fibres) in the lungs are indicative of exposure, but not disease. The type and extent of disease largely depend on exposure. **Asbestosis** is a fibrotic lung disease developing up to 10 years after heavy exposure. Patients present with progressive dyspnoea, basal crackles on inspiration and sometimes finger clubbing. There is a restrictive lung function defect and reduced D_LCO, with diffuse streaky shadows on X-ray and thickening of visceral pleura; **honeycomb lung** is often prominent in the lower lobes. Prognosis is poor. **Mesothelioma** (Chapter 34) can develop up to 40 years after light exposure, and is invariably fatal. Milder forms of asbestos-induced pleural disease produce dyspnoea and restrictive defects coupled with pleural thickening and plaques or effusions, with scattered fibrotic foci. No treatment is effective for asbestos-related disease, as the stimulus remains in the lungs. Asbestos-related lung cancer is discussed in Chapter 42.

Silicosis is a fibrotic disease caused by inhalation of silica, with a low prevalence in developed nations. Occupations at risk include mining, stone working, manufacture of abrasives, foundry work and glass working. Silica is very toxic to macrophages and thus highly fibrogenic. Chronic silicosis (over decades) is characterized by **silicotic nodules** of collagen around a cell-free core, first developing in hilar lymph nodes. In acute silicosis due to heavy exposure, severe dyspnoea may develop over months. The clinical features of silicosis are similar to PMF.

Inhalation of organic material

Extrinsic allergic alveolitis (or **hypersensitivity pneumonitis**) is a diffuse inflammatory disease of small airways and alveoli caused by allergens, primarily microbial spores, that are small enough to reach the alveoli (Fig. 35b). The most common example is **farmer's lung**, caused by dust from mouldy hay or plants contaminated with **thermophilic actinomycetes** bacteria, which thrive in warm moist conditions. Typically, symptoms occur several hours after exposure, and include fever, dyspnoea and cough. Although early removal of exposure results in rapid recovery, continuous exposure leads to progressive **interstitial fibrosis** (Chapter 32), with infiltration of inflammatory cells and formation of **granulomas** (chronically inflamed tissue masses characterized by multinucleate giant cells, see Fig. 29b). Patients present with dyspnoea, restrictive defects and decreased D_LCO. Fluffy nodular shadowing or ground glass opacity may be shown in CXR, with honeycomb lung (Chapter 32) in severe cases. Detailed histories are required to establish probable antigens, with confirmation by detection of precipitating antibodies in serum. **Management** centres on abolishing antigen exposure. High-dose corticosteroids can regress early disease, but established disease with fibrosis is irreversible and can progress to respiratory failure. **Differential diagnosis** includes asthma (Chapters 26 and 27), sarcoidosis (Chapter 33), viral and mycoplasma pneumonias (Chapters 38 and 39) and mycobacterial infections.

Byssinosis occurs in workers handling raw cotton, flax and hemp. It is characterized by chest tightness, cough and/or shortness of breath on the first day back at work, with recovery as the week progresses. It is primarily due to acute bronchoconstriction, possibly related to contaminating bacterial endotoxins. Long-term exposure causes a disease similar to chronic bronchitis (Chapter 28), with chronic productive cough, progressive decline in lung function and disability.

36 Cystic fibrosis and bronchiectasis

Figure 36a Mean survival of CF patients

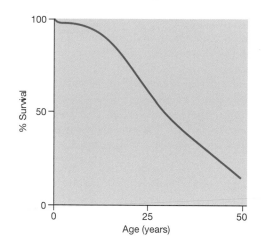

Figure 36b Development of respiratory problems in CF

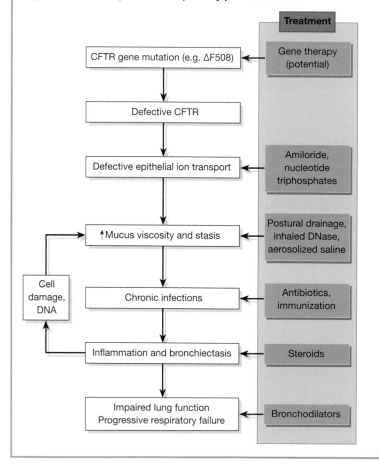

Figure 36c Other conditions associated with CF

Condition	% of CF patents
Delayed development, puberty	100%
Male infertility (absent/obstructed vas deferens and epididymis)	98%
Female infertility	20%
Pancreatic insufficiency	85%
Nasal polyps	15–20%, most in 2nd decade
Symptomatic sinusitis	10% children 25% adults
Rectal prolapse	20% children Rare in adults
Bone demineralization (vitamin D deficiency)	Common
Hypertrophic osteoarthropathy	15% adults
Dysfunctional gallbladder or gallstones	10–30%
Biliary cirrhosis	5% adults

Figure 36d Some conditions associated with bronchiectasis

- Allergic bronchopulmonary aspergillosis (Chapter 35)
- α_1-Antitrypsin deficiency (Chapters 19 and 28)
- Bronchial obstruction (foreign bodies, mucus, tumour)
- Congenital cartilage deficiency (Williams–Campbell syndrome)
- **Cystic fibrosis**
- Fibrotic disease and alveolitis (Chapters 32 and 35)
- HIV and immunodeficiency (Chapter 41)
- Infection (e.g. measles and pertussis), pneumonia (Chapters 38 and 39)
- Lung transplant
- Primary ciliary dyskinesia (Kartagener's syndrome, Chapter 19)
- Rheumatoid arthritis
- Tuberculosis (Chapter 40)
- Tracheobronchomegaly (Mounier–Kuhn syndrome)

The Respiratory System at a Glance, Fourth Edition. Jeremy P.T. Ward. © Jeremy P.T. Ward. Published 2015 by John Wiley & Sons, Ltd.

Cystic fibrosis (CF) is the primary cause of severe chronic lung disease in children, although 90% of children now survive into their second decade (Fig. 36a). CF is characterized by **chronic bronchopulmonary infection** and airway obstruction (Fig. 36b) and by **exocrine pancreatic insufficiency** with consequent effects on gut function, nutrition and development. The key feature of CF is **increased viscosity** and **subsequent stasis of epithelial mucus**. There is usually an **increased salt content of sweat**. Figure 36c shows some associated disorders.

CF is an **autosomal recessive trait** that is the most common genetic cause of morbidity and mortality in the white population, with a prevalence of approximately 1 in 2000 live births; nearly 5% of white people of European descent are heterozygous carriers. Prevalence is far less in others, being approximately 1 in 17,000 for those of African descent. CF is due to mutations in a gene on chromosome 7 encoding for the **cystic fibrosis transmembrane conductance regulator** (CFTR), a cAMP-regulated epithelial chloride channel that can also alter activity of other ionic transporters. Dysfunction of CFTR impairs epithelial chloride, sodium and water transfer and thus causes **reduced mucus hydration** and **increased viscosity** (Chapter 21). Over 800 mutations in the CFTR gene have been described, but the most common, found in approximately 65% of patients with CF, is deletion of the phenylalanine codon at position 508, the **ΔF508** mutation.

Clinical features

The lungs of neonates with CF are often normal, but rapid development of respiratory symptoms, including refractory cough and infections, is usual. CF patients nearly always have an increased lung volume and **finger clubbing** (increased curvature of the nail and loss of normal angle between nail and nail bed) (Chapter 21). Recurrent bronchopulmonary infections, primarily as a result of defective mucus clearance, are rarely cleared once established and eventually result in **bronchiectasis** (see below), extensive lung damage and dysfunction. Spontaneous **pneumothorax** (Chapter 37) and **haemoptysis** (spitting blood; Case 5 [or Case 5 online]) are not uncommon. About 10% of neonates present with meconium ileus (failure to pass meconium), which can cause death in the first day of life; 20% of older patients exhibit a similar ileal obstruction (**meconium ileus equivalent**, MIE). Eighty-five per cent of patients have steatorrhoea (high-fat stools) as a result of pancreatic insufficiency. Some patients have only mild respiratory symptoms for many years, but this is inevitably followed by a characteristic increase in the frequency and severity of exacerbation of symptoms (cough, dyspnoea, loss of appetite). Eventually, severe restrictions in activity herald the end-stage disease, followed by respiratory failure, hypoxaemia, pulmonary hypertension and death.

Diagnosis

Several factors need to be taken into account, including a **family history** of the disease and the presence of typical respiratory and gastrointestinal disorders (Fig. 36c). A **sweat chloride** or **sodium** concentration above 60 mmol/L is diagnostic when coupled with such disorders, although approximately 1% of CF patients may have normal sweat electrolytes. DNA analysis can detect known mutations (e.g. ΔF508), but is limited by the high number of unknown mutations. In later disease, chest X-rays can detect bronchiectasis (see below). Neonates can be screened for CF by blood immunoreactive trypsin, which can detect many, but not all cases.

Management

The primary objectives of treatment are to **control infection, promote mucus clearance** and **improve nutrition**. Early antibiotic therapy is crucial to inhibit progression. Choice of antibiotic is determined by the infecting organisms. The dosage should be higher in CF patients and the course longer. Development of resistance is a key problem and is transferable; segregation of patients is thus advisable. Immunization for measles, pertussis and influenza is important, as these are particularly dangerous in CF. Bronchodilators (β-agonists) may improve lung function, and corticosteroids may assist inflammation in some patients.

Clearance: Training by physiotherapists in postural drainage (tipping the body so that the infected lobe is uppermost) is vital, coupled with chest percussion to mobilize secretions to the upper airways where they can be coughed up. Such treatment is prescribed one to four times a day. Recently introduced therapies include inhalation of DNase, an enzyme that breaks down DNA from dead cells, which contributes to mucus viscosity. Inhalation of aerosolized saline may improve mucus hydration, as may blockade of sodium reabsorption with amiloride or stimulation of chloride secretion with nucleotide triphosphates. Cough should never be suppressed, as it is an important method of clearance.

Novel therapies: Ivacaftor, which potentiates CFTR opening, was recently approved for patients 6+ years old with the G551D mutation (~4% cases). It is ineffective for ΔF508 which prevents insertion of CFTR into the membrane. Recent trials with ivacaftor in combination with VX-809, a "corrector" that moves defective CFTR to the membrane, have however been promising.

Nutrition: Most patients with CF require pancreatic enzymes with meals, supplemented with vitamins. High-calorific foods should be advised.

Bronchiectasis

Bronchiectasis is an abnormal and permanent dilatation of proximal (>2 mm) bronchi due to inflammation and subsequent destruction of the elastic and muscular components of their walls (Case 5 [or Case 5 online]). It is normally associated with defects in **mucociliary clearance** (Chapter 19) and **persistent respiratory infections**. Onset is often in childhood, following pulmonary infections complicating measles or pertussis. Since the introduction of antibiotics, the most common cause of bronchiectasis is CF (Fig. 36d), except in poorly resourced countries. Symptoms depend on the severity and location of diseased bronchi, but commonly include persistent productive cough, with large quantities of foul-smelling purulent sputum as the disease worsens. Severity has been correlated with the volume of sputum produced, but not with dyspnoea. Haemoptysis and recurrent pneumonia or abscesses are common; haemoptysis is normally mild, but can become life-threatening, particularly in CF patients. Fever, anaemia and weight loss may accompany the disease. Patients often develop finger clubbing, metastatic abscesses, respiratory failure and amyloidosis. Chest X-rays and high-resolution computed tomography (HRCT) can often detect the dilated and thickened bronchi (Case 5). **Management** is similar to that for CF, although without the nutritional requirements.

37 Pneumothorax

Figure 37a Pneumothorax

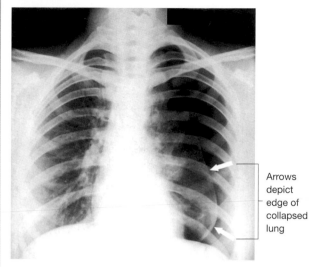

Arrows depict edge of collapsed lung

Small pneumothorax

<30%

Moderate pneumothorax

>30%

Complete pneumothorax

Tension pneumothorax

Compressed lung

Deviated trachea

Mediastinal shift

Figure 37b Pneumothorax management

Type of pneumothorax	Degree of collapse		
	Complete	Moderate	Small
Primary	Aspirate/chest drain	Aspirate	Observe
Secondary	Chest drain	Chest drain	Chest drain
Traumatic/Iatrogenic	Chest drain	Chest drain	Observe/chest drain

Figure 37d Seldinger technique for insertion of a chest drain

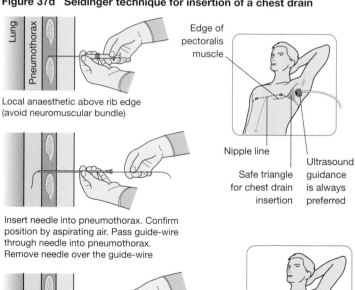

Local anaesthetic above rib edge (avoid neuromuscular bundle)

Insert needle into pneumothorax. Confirm position by aspirating air. Pass guide-wire through needle into pneumothorax. Remove needle over the guide-wire

Pass dilator over the wire. Then remove dilator

Pass drain over wire. Then remove the wire. Position drain in lung apex. Then stitch the drain in place

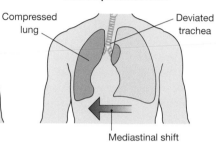

Edge of pectoralis muscle

Nipple line

Safe triangle for chest drain insertion

Ultrasound guidance is always preferred

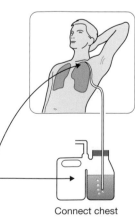

Connect chest drain to an underwater seal

Figure 37c Aspiration

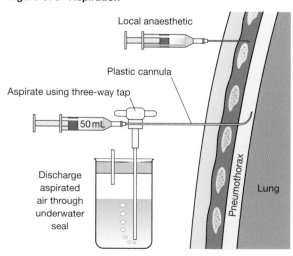

Local anaesthetic

Plastic cannula

Aspirate using three-way tap

50 mL

Discharge aspirated air through underwater seal

Pneumothorax

Lung

The Respiratory System at a Glance, Fourth Edition. Jeremy P.T. Ward. © Jeremy P.T. Ward. Published 2015 by John Wiley & Sons, Ltd.

Apneumothorax is a collection of air between the visceral and parietal pleura causing a real rather than potential pleural space. Recognition and early drainage can be lifesaving. Predisposing and precipitating factors include necrotizing lung pathology, chest trauma, ventilator-associated lung injury and cardiothoracic surgery.

Pneumothorax classification

Primary spontaneous pneumothorax

This is caused by rupture of small apical subpleural air cysts ('blebs') but rarely causes significant physiological disturbance. Tall young (20–40 years old) men (male/female 5:1) with no underlying lung disease are usually affected. It is the most common type of pneumothorax (prevalence 8/10^5 per year, rising to 200/10^5 per year in subjects >1.9 m in height). Following a second primary spontaneous pneumothorax (PSP), recurrence is likely (>60%) and pleurodesis to fuse the visceral and parietal pleura using medical (e.g. pleural insertion of talc) or surgical (e.g. abrasion of the pleural) means is recommended.

Secondary pneumothorax

This is associated with respiratory diseases that damage lung architecture, most commonly obstructive (e.g. chronic obstructive pulmonary disease (COPD) and asthma), fibrotic or infective (e.g. pneumonia), and occasionally rare or inherited disorders (e.g. Marfan's and cystic fibrosis). The incidence of secondary pneumothorax (SP) increases with age and the severity of the underlying lung disease. These patients usually require hospital admission as even a small SP in a patient with reduced respiratory reserve may have more serious implications than a large PSP. ICU patients with lung disease are at particular risk of SP due to the high pressures ('barotrauma') and alveolar overdistention ('volutrauma') associated with mechanical ventilation. 'Protective' ventilation strategies using low-pressure, limited volume ventilation reduce this risk.

Traumatic (iatrogenic) pneumothorax

This follows blunt (e.g. road traffic accidents) or penetrating (e.g. fractured ribs and stab wounds) chest trauma. Therapeutic procedures (e.g. line insertion and thoracic surgery) are common causes of iatrogenic pneumothorax.

Tension pneumothorax

A **tension pneumothorax** may complicate PSP or SP but is most common during mechanical ventilation and following traumatic pneumothorax. It occurs when air accumulates in the pleural cavity faster than it can be removed. Increased intrathoracic pressure causes mediastinal shift, compression of functioning lung, inhibition of venous return and shock due to reduced cardiac output. It is a medical emergency and fatal if not rapidly relieved by drainage. Detection is a clinical diagnosis; awaiting chest X-ray (CXR) confirmation may be life-threatening. Immediate drainage with a 14G needle in the second intercostal space in the midclavicular line is essential. A characteristic 'hiss' of escaping gas confirms the diagnosis. A chest drain is then inserted.

Clinical assessment

Pneumothorax is graded and treated according to Figures 37a and 37b. Sudden breathlessness and/or sharp pleuritic pain suggests a pneumothorax. Most PSPs are small (<30%) and cause few symptoms other than pain. Clinical signs can be surprisingly difficult to detect, but in larger pneumothoraxes reduced air entry and hyperresonant percussion over one hemithorax are characteristic and may be associated with tachypnoea and cyanosis. Cardiorespiratory compromise may develop remarkably

quickly in a tension pneumothorax and requires immediate drainage. Occasionally, other pulmonary air leaks may occur (see below). **Monitoring** reveals tachycardia, hypotension and desaturation. **Blood gases** may demonstrate respiratory failure. CXR confirms the diagnosis (Fig. 37a). **Computed tomography (CT) scan** may detect localized pneumothoraxes.

Management

Immediate supportive therapy includes supplemental oxygen and analgesia. Treatment is dependent on the cause, size and symptoms.

A tension pneumothorax must be drained immediately. A small PSP (<30%; <2 cm between lung edge and chest wall at hilar level) is simply observed and spontaneous reabsorption is confirmed on serial outpatient CXR. A PSP >30% (>2 cm between lung edge and chest wall) may be aspirated through a 16–18G needle in the second intercostal space in the midclavicular line, using a 50 mL syringe connected to a three-way tap and underwater seal (Fig. 37c). Following overnight observation, successful aspiration is confirmed by lung re-expansion on repeat CXR. Occasionally, intercostal tube drainage is required for a large PSP with respiratory failure or if aspiration is unsuccessful.

In general, SP and traumatic pneumothoraxes *always* require hospital admission and intercostal chest drain insertion. The 'Seldinger' technique (i.e. chest drain inserted over a guide wire) is commonly employed but can be associated with complications and if possible insertion should be performed during daytime hours under mandatory ultrasound guidance (Fig. 37d). In difficult cases a chest drain can be inserted using the relatively safe 'blunt dissection' technique. Small chest drains (16G) are nearly always adequate. Large chest drains are painful and have no significant benefits. In mechanically ventilated patients, high airway pressures or large tidal volumes encourage persistent leaks and must be avoided.

A persistent drain leak suggests development of a **bronchopleural fistula** (BPF). High flow, wall suction with pressures of 5–50 cmH_2O, may oppose visceral and parietal pleura, allowing spontaneous pleurodesis. Physiotherapy and bronchial toilette are required to maintain airway patency. Early advice on surgical BPF management is essential. Video-assisted thoracoscopy is as effective as thoracotomy at correcting BPF but causes less respiratory dysfunction.

Chest drains are removed when CXR confirms lung expansion and there has been no air leakage through the drain for more than 24 hours. Drains should not be clamped before removal. Following adequate analgesia, the drain is pulled out when the patient is in inspiration. Purse string sutures around the drainage site are then tightly secured.

Air leaks

Pneumomediastinum describes air in the mediastinal–pleural reflection, outlining the heart and great vessels on CXR. Air may also dissect along perivascular sheaths into the neck, causing **subcutaneous emphysema (SE)** or around the heart with **pneumopericardium**, which may cause tamponade. Air leaks follow traumatic damage to the trachea, bronchus and oesophagus or ventilator-induced barotrauma. SE may cause localized cervical or grotesque facial and body swelling. It has a characteristic crackling sensation on palpation. The voice may have a nasal quality, and auscultation over the precordium may reveal a 'crunch' with each heart beat (Homan's sign). Management includes good drainage of pneumothorax and 'protective' ventilation strategies (Chapter 44). Failure of spontaneous resolution should prompt investigation, including bronchoscopy, for problems that decrease chest drain efficiency or undetected air leaks.

38 Community-acquired pneumonia

Figure 38a Pneumonia affecting the right lower lobe

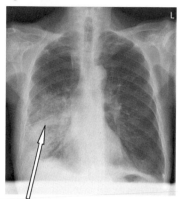

Consolidation right lower lobe

Figure 38b Pneumonia affecting lingula lobe

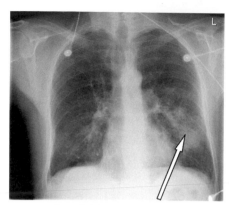

Consolidation lingula lobe

Table 1 Risk factors for pneumonia

Age: >65, <5 years old
Chronic disease (e.g. renal and lung)
Diabetes mellitus
Immunosuppression (e.g. drugs and HIV)
Alcohol dependency
Aspiration (e.g. epilepsy)
Recent viral illness (e.g. influenza)
Malnutrition
Mechanical ventilation
Postoperative (e.g. obesity and smoking)
Environmental (e.g. psittacosis)
Occupational (e.g. Q fever)
Travel abroad (e.g. paragonimiasis)
Air conditioning (e.g. *Legionella*)

Table 2 Microorganisms and pathological insults that cause pneumonia

Bacterial infections	Atypical infections	Fungal infection
Streptococcus pneumoniae *Haemophilus influenzae* *Klebsiella pneumoniae* *Pseudomonas aeruginosa* Gram-negative (*E. coli*)	*Mycoplasma pneumoniae* *Legionella pneumophila* *Coxiella burnetii* *Chlamydia psittaci*	*Aspergillus* *Histoplasmosis* *Candida* *Nocardia*
Viral infections	**Protozoal infections**	**Other causes**
Influenza Coxsackie Adenovirus Respiratory syncytial Cytomegalovirus	*Pneumocystis carinii* Toxoplasmosis Amoebiasis Paragonimiasis	Aspiration Lipoid pneumonia Bronchiectasis Cystic fibrosis Radiation

Figure 38.3 Non-hospital (i.e. community) management of CAP using the recently validated CRB-65 score

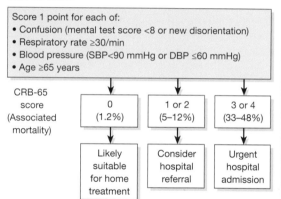

Score 1 point for each of:
• Confusion (mental test score <8 or new disorientation)
• Respiratory rate ≥30/min
• Blood pressure (SBP<90 mmHg or DBP ≤60 mmHg)
• Age ≥65 years

CRB-65 score (Associated mortality)

0 (1.2%)	1 or 2 (5–12%)	3 or 4 (33–48%)
Likely suitable for home treatment	Consider hospital referral	Urgent hospital admission

Figure 38.5 Complications and infection specific features of pneumonia

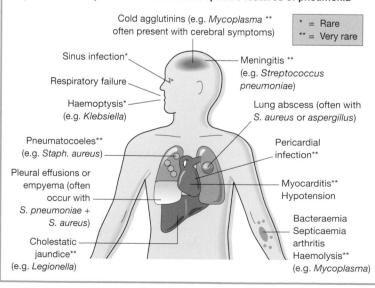

Cold agglutinins (e.g. *Mycoplasma* ** often present with cerebral symptoms)

* = Rare
** = Very rare

Sinus infection*

Meningitis ** (e.g. *Streptococcus pneumoniae*)

Respiratory failure

Haemoptysis* (e.g. *Klebsiella*)

Lung abscess (often with *S. aureus* or *aspergillus*)

Pneumatocoeles** (e.g. *Staph. aureus*)

Pericardial infection**

Pleural effusions or empyema (often occur with *S. pneumoniae* + *S. aureus*)

Myocarditis** Hypotension

Bacteraemia Septicaemia arthritis Haemolysis** (e.g. *Mycoplasma*)

Cholestatic jaundice** (e.g. *Legionella*)

Figure 38.2 Management of CAP in patients admitted to hospital using the recently validated CURB-65 score

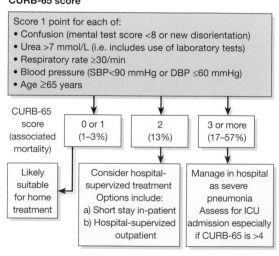

Score 1 point for each of:
• Confusion (mental test score <8 or new disorientation)
• Urea >7 mmol/L (i.e. includes use of laboratory tests)
• Respiratory rate ≥30/min
• Blood pressure (SBP<90 mmHg or DBP ≤60 mmHg)
• Age ≥65 years

CURB-65 score (associated mortality)

0 or 1 (1–3%)	2 (13%)	3 or more (17–57%)
Likely suitable for home treatment	Consider hospital-supervized treatment Options include: a) Short stay in-patient b) Hospital-supervized outpatient	Manage in hospital as severe pneumonia Assess for ICU admission especially if CURB-65 is >4

The Respiratory System at a Glance, Fourth Edition. Jeremy P.T. Ward. © Jeremy P.T. Ward. Published 2015 by John Wiley & Sons, Ltd.

Pneumonia is an acute lower respiratory tract (LRT) illness, usually due to infection, associated with fever, focal chest symptoms (± signs) and new shadowing on chest X-ray (CXR) (Fig. 38a). Table 1 lists causes of pneumonia.

Classification

Microbiological classification of pneumonia is not practical as causative organisms may not be identified or diagnosis takes several days. Likewise, radiographic appearance (e.g. lobar- (i.e. one lobe) or bronchopneumonia (i.e. widespread, patchy involvement)) gives little information about cause. The following classification is widely accepted.

- **Community-acquired pneumonia (CAP):** describes LRT infections occurring before or within 48 hours of hospital admission in patients who have not been hospitalized for >14 days. The most frequently identified organism is *Streptococcus pneumoniae* (20–75%). Atypical pathogens (e.g. *Mycoplasma pneumoniae*, *Chlamydia pneumonia*, *Legionella* spp: 2–25%) and viral infections (8–12%) are relatively common causes. *Haemophilus influenzae* and *Moraxella catarrhalis* occur in COPD exacerbations and staphylococcal infections may follow influenza. Alcoholic, diabetic and nursing-home patients are prone to staphylococcal, anaerobic and Gram-negative organisms.
- **Hospital-acquired (nosocomial) pneumonia** (Chapter 39): LRT infections developing >2 days after hospital admission. Likely organisms are Gram-negative bacilli (~70%) or staphylococci (~15%).
- **Aspiration/anaerobic pneumonia:** bacteroides and other anaerobic infections follow aspiration of oropharyngeal contents (e.g. CVA).
- **Opportunistic pneumonia** (Chapter 39): immunosuppressed patients (e.g. chemotherapy, HIV) are susceptible to viral, fungal, mycobacterial and unusual bacterial infections.
- **Recurrent pneumonia:** is due to aerobic and anaerobic organisms in cystic fibrosis and bronchiectasis.

Epidemiology

Annual incidence: 5–11 cases per 1000 adult population; 15–45% require hospitalization of whom 5–10% are treated in ICU. Incidence is highest in the elderly and infants. **Mortality:** 6–12% in hospitalized and 25–>50% in ICU patients. **Seasonal variation:** (e.g. *Mycoplasma* in autumn, *Staphylococcus* in spring) and annual cycles (e.g. 4-yearly *Mycoplasma* epidemics). Viral infections increase CAP in winter.

Risk factors

Factors increasing CAP risk are listed in Table 2. **Specific factors** include **age** (e.g. *Mycoplasma* in young adults); **occupation** (e.g. brucellosis in abattoir workers, Q fever in sheep workers); **environment** (e.g. psittacosis with pet birds); or **geographical** (e.g. coccidioidomycosis in southwest USA). Epidemics of *Coxiella burnetii* (Q fever) or *Legionella pneumophila* may be localized (e.g. Legionnaire's disease may involve a specific hotel due to air-conditioner contamination).

Diagnosis

The aims are to establish the **diagnosis**, identify **complications**, assess **severity** and determine **classification** to aid antibiotic choice.

Clinical features

These are not diagnostic without a CXR and cannot predict causative organisms (i.e. 'atypical' pathogens do not have characteristic presentations). **Symptoms** may be general (e.g. malaise, fever, myalgia) or chest specific (e.g. dyspnoea, pleurisy, cough, haemoptysis). **Signs** include cyanosis, tachycardia and tachypnoea; with focal dullness, crepitations, bronchial breathing and pleuritic rub on chest examination. In the young, elderly and atypical pneumonias (e.g. *Mycoplasma*), **non-respiratory features** (e.g. confusion, rashes, diarrhoea) may predominate. **Complications** are shown in Figure 38e.

Investigations

Blood tests: white cell count (WCC) and C-reactive protein confirm infection; haemolysis and cold agglutinins occur in ~50% of *Mycoplasma* infection; abnormal liver function tests suggest *Legionella* or *Mycoplasma* infection. **Blood gases:** identify respiratory failure. **Microbiology:** no organism is isolated in ~33–50% of patients due to previous antibiotic therapy or poor specimen collection. Blood cultures, sputum, pleural fluid and bronchoalveolar lavage samples, with appropriate staining, culture and assessment of antibiotic sensitivity, determines the pathogen and effective therapy. **Serology:** identifies *Mycoplasma* infection but long processing times limit clinical value. Rapid antigen detection for *Legionella* (e.g. urine) and pneumococcus (e.g. serum, pleural fluid) is more useful. **Radiology:** CXR (Fig. 38a) and CT scans aid diagnosis and detect complications.

Severity assessment

Features associated with increased mortality and the need for ICU monitoring are: **Clinical:** age >60 years; respiratory rate >30/min; diastolic blood pressure <60 mmHg; new atrial fibrillation; confusion; multilobar involvement; and coexisting illness; **Laboratory:** urea >7 mmol/L; albumin <35 g/L; hypoxaemia Po_2 <8 kPa; leukopenia (WCC <4 × 10^9/L); leucocytosis (WCC >20 × 10^9/L); and bacteraemia. **Severity scoring:** CRB-65 and CURB-65 scores, allocate points for **c**onfusion; **u**rea >7 mmol/L; **r**espiratory rate >30/min; low systolic (<90 mmHg) or diastolic (<60 mmHg) **b**lood pressure and age >**65** years, to stratify patients into mortality groups and appropriate management pathways (Figs. 38c and 38d).

Management

Supportive measures: include oxygen to maintain P_aO_2 >8 kPa (S_aO_2 <90%) and intravenous fluid (± inotrope) resuscitation to ensure haemodynamic stability. **Ventilatory support:** consider non-invasive or mechanical ventilation in respiratory failure (Chapter 44). **Physiotherapy and bronchoscopy:** aid sputum clearance.

Initial antibiotic therapy: represents the 'best guess', according to pneumonia classification and likely organisms, as microbiological results are not available for 12–72 hours. Therapy is adjusted when results and antibiotic sensitivities are available. The American and British Thoracic Societies (ATS, BTS) recommend the following initial antibiotic protocols for CAP:

- **Non-hospitalized patients:** are treated with oral amoxicillin (BTS) or a macrolide (e.g. clarithromycin) or doxycycline (ATS). Patients with severe symptoms or at risk for drug-resistant *S. pneumoniae* (e.g. recent antibiotics, comorbidity) require a β-lactam plus a macrolide or doxycycline; or an antipneumococcal fluoroquinolone (e.g. moxifloxacin) alone.
- **Hospitalized patients:** initial therapy must cover both 'atypical' organisms and *S. pneumoniae*. An intravenous macrolide is combined with a β-lactam or an antipneumococcal fluoroquinolone (ATS/BTS) or cefuroxime (BTS). If not severe, combined ampicillin and macrolide (oral) is adequate (BTS). Cover staphylococcal infection after influenza and *H. influenzae* in COPD.

39 Hospital-acquired (nosocomial) pneumonia

Figure 39a (i) CXR; (ii) CT scan from a patient with hospital-acquired pneumonia (HAP) showing consolidation, cavitation and abscess formation

(i)

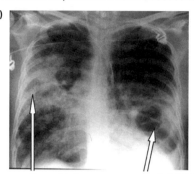

Consolidation   Cavitation

Fluid-filled abscess

(ii)

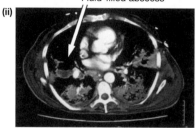

Table 2 Risk factors for multidrug-resistant pathogens causing hospital-acquired pneumonia

- Antimicrobial therapy in the previous 90 days
- Current hospitalization of >5 days
- High frequency of local antibiotic resistance
- Presence of risk factors for HCAP
  - hospitalization for >2 days in the previous 90 days
  - residence in a nursing home
  - home wound care or intravenous therapy
  - chronic dialysis within 30 days
  - family member with MDR pathogen
- Immunosuppressive disease and/or therapy

Table 1 Risk factors and modifiable risk factors for HAP and VAP

Unmodifiable risk factors	Modifiable risk factors
1. Host related • Malnutrition • Age: >65, <5 years old • Chronic disease (e.g. renal) • Diabetes • Immunosuppression (e.g. SLE) • Alcohol dependency • Aspiration (e.g. epilepsy) • Recent viral illness • Obesity • Smoking **2. Therapy related** • Mechanical ventilation • Postoperative	**1. Host related** • Nutrition • Pain control, physiotherapy • Limit immunosuppressive therapy • Posture • Preoperative smoking cessation **2. Therapy related** • Semi-recumbent position • Early removal of iv lines, ET and NG tubes • minimize sedative use • Avoid gastric overdistention • Avoid re-intubation • Change ventilator circuits **3. Infection control** • Hand washing, sterile technique • Patient isolation • Microbiological surveillance

Figure 39b Pathogenesis of hospital aquired pneumonia

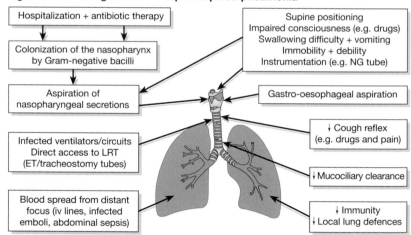

Hospitalization + antibiotic therapy

Colonization of the nasopharynx by Gram-negative bacilli

Aspiration of nasopharyngeal secretions

Infected ventilators/circuits Direct access to LRT (ET/tracheostomy tubes)

Blood spread from distant focus (iv lines, infected emboli, abdominal sepsis)

Supine positioning
Impaired consciousness (e.g. drugs)
Swallowing difficulty + vomiting
Immobility + debility
Instrumentation (e.g. NG tube)

Gastro-oesophageal aspiration

↓ Cough reflex (e.g. drugs and pain)

↓ Mucociliary clearance

↓ Immunity
↓ Local lung defences

Figure 39c Likely pathogens and empirical antibiotic treatment of hospital-acquired pneumonias

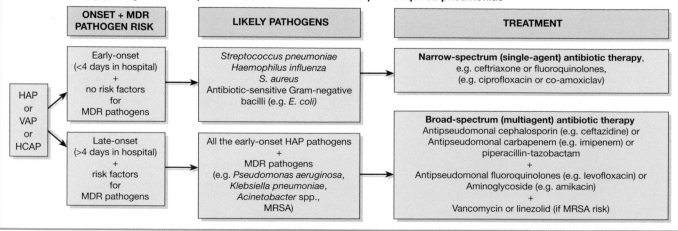

ONSET + MDR PATHOGEN RISK	LIKELY PATHOGENS	TREATMENT
HAP or VAP or HCAP → Early-onset (<4 days in hospital) + no risk factors for MDR pathogens	*Streptococcus pneumoniae* *Haemophilus influenza* *S. aureus* Antibiotic-sensitive Gram-negative bacilli (e.g. *E. coli*)	**Narrow-spectrum (single-agent) antibiotic therapy,** e.g. ceftriaxone or fluoroquinolones, (e.g. ciprofloxacin or co-amoxiclav)
Late-onset (>4 days in hospital) + risk factors for MDR pathogens	All the early-onset HAP pathogens + MDR pathogens (e.g. *Pseudomonas aeruginosa*, *Klebsiella pneumoniae*, *Acinetobacter* spp., MRSA)	**Broad-spectrum (multiagent) antibiotic therapy** Antipseudomonal cephalosporin (e.g. ceftazidine) or Antipseudomonal carbapenem (e.g. imipenem) or piperacillin-tazobactam + Antipseudomonal fluoroquinolones (e.g. levofloxacin) or Aminoglycoside (e.g. amikacin) + Vancomycin or linezolid (if MRSA risk)

The Respiratory System at a Glance, Fourth Edition. Jeremy P.T. Ward. © Jeremy P.T. Ward. Published 2015 by John Wiley & Sons, Ltd.

Hospital-acquired (nosocomial) pneumonia (HAP) including ventilator-associated pneumonia (VAP) and healthcare-associated pneumonia (HCAP) affects 0.5–2% of hospital patients. It is a major cause of nosocomial infection (i.e. with wound, urinary tract, blood stream). Pathogenesis, causative organisms and outcome differ from community-acquired pneumonia (CAP). Prevention, early antibiotic therapy and an awareness of the role of multidrug resistant (MDR) pathogens, improves outcome.

Definitions

HAP is pulmonary infection that develops >48 hours after hospital admission that was not incubating at the time of admission. VAP is pneumonia developing >48–72 hours after endotracheal intubation. HCAP includes patients residing in nursing homes, receiving therapy (e.g. wound care, intravenous therapy) within 30 days or admitted to hospital for >2 days within 90 days of the current infection or attending a hospital or haemodialysis clinic.

Epidemiology

Incidence: varies between 5–10 episodes per 1000 discharges and is highest on surgical and ICU wards and in teaching hospitals. It lengthens hospital stay by 3–14 days per patient. The risk of HAP increases 6–20-fold during mechanical ventilation (MV) and in ICU, is responsible for 25% of infections and ~50% of prescribed antibiotics. VAP accounts for >80% of HAP and occurs in 9–27% of intubated patients. Risk factors: include CAP risk factors and those associated with HAP pathogenesis, some of which can be prevented (Table 1). Mortality is between 30% and 70%. Early onset HAP/VAP (<4 days in hospital) is usually caused by antibiotic-sensitive bacteria and carries a better prognosis than late onset HAP/VAP (>4 days in hospital), which is associated with MDR pathogens. In early onset HAP/VAP, prior antibiotic therapy or hospitalization predisposes to MDR pathogens and is treated as late onset HAP/VAP. Bacteraemia, medical rather than surgical illness, VAP and late or ineffective antibiotic therapy increases mortality.

Pathogenesis

The oropharynx is colonized by enteric Gram-negative bacteria in most hospital patients due to immobility, impaired consciousness, instrumentation (e.g. nasogastric tubes), poor hygiene or inhibition of gastric acid secretion. Subsequent aspiration of oral secretions (± gastric contents) causes HAP (Fig. 39b).

Aetiology

Early or late onset and risk factors for infection with MDR organisms (Table 2) determine likely pathogens (Fig. 39c). Aerobic Gram-negative bacilli (e.g. *Klebsiella pneumoniae*, *Pseudomonas aeruginosa*, *Escherichia coli*) cause ~60–70% and *Staphylococcus aureus* ~10–15% of infections. *Streptococcus pneumoniae* and *Haemophilus influenza* may be isolated in early onset HAP/VAP. In ICU, >50% *S. aureus* infections are methicillin resistant (MRSA). *S. aureus* is more common in diabetics and ICU patients.

Diagnosis

Requires both *clinical* and *microbiological* assessment. Non-specific clinical features, concurrent illness (e.g. ARDS); and previous antibiotics which limit microbiological evaluation can make diagnosis difficult. Clinical: suspect HAP when new CXR infiltrates occur with features suggestive of infection (e.g. fever >38°C, purulent sputum, leucocytosis, hypoxaemia). Diagnostic tests: confirm infection and establish the causative organism (± antibiotic sensitivity). They include blood counts and gases, serology, blood cultures, pleural fluid and endotracheal aspirates, sputum, bronchoalveolar lavage, and CXR. CT scans (Fig. 39a.ii.) aid diagnosis and detect complications (e.g. abscesses).

Management

Early diagnosis and treatment improves morbidity and mortality. Do not delay antibiotic therapy whilst awaiting microbiological results.

Supportive therapy

Supplemental oxygen maintains P_aO_2 >8 kPa (S_aO_2 <90%), intravenous fluids (± inotropes) preserve haemodynamic stability and ventilatory support (e.g. CPAP, MV) corrects respiratory failure. Physiotherapy and analgesia aid sputum clearance postoperatively and in immobilized patients. Semi-recumbent (i.e. 30° bed-head elevation) nursing of bed-bound patients reduces aspiration risk. Strict glycaemic control and attention to other modifiable risk factors (Table 1) may improve outcome.

Antibiotic therapy

This is empirical while awaiting microbiological guidance. The key factor is whether the patient is at risk of MDR organisms. Figure 39c illustrates the ATS guidelines for initial, i.v. antibiotic therapy. Local patterns of antibiotic resistance are used to modify these protocols.

• In early onset HAP/VAP with no risk factors for MDR organisms, use monotherapy with a β-lactam/β-lactamase, third-generation cephalosporin or fluoroquinolone antibiotic.
• In late onset HAP/VAP with risk factors for MDR pathogens (Table 2), start combination therapy (Fig. 39c) with broad-spectrum antibiotics to cover MDR Gram-negative bacilli and MRSA (e.g. vancomycin). Consider adjunctive therapy with inhaled aminoglycosides or polymyxin in patients not improving with systemic therapy.

A short course of therapy (e.g. 7 days) is appropriate if the clinical response is good. Resistant pathogens (e.g. *P. aeruginosa*, *S. aureus*) may require 14–21 days' treatment. Focus therapy on causative organisms when culture data are available and withdraw unnecessary antibiotics. Sterile cultures (without new antibiotics for >72 hours) virtually rule out HAP.

Other pneumonias

Aspiration/anaerobic pneumonia: anaerobic infection (e.g. Bacteroides) follows aspiration of oropharyngeal contents due to laryngeal incompetence or reduced consciousness (e.g. CVA, drugs). Lung abscesses are common. Antibiotic therapy should include anaerobic coverage (e.g. metronidazole).

Pneumonia during immunosuppression (Chapter 41): HIV, transplant and chemotherapy patients are susceptible to viral (e.g. cytomegalovirus), fungal (e.g. *Aspergillus*) and mycobacterial infections. HIV patients with CD4 counts <200/mm^3, may also develop opportunistic infections such as *Pneumocystis jirovecii (carinii)* pneumonia (PCP) or toxoplasma. Severely immunocompromised patients require broad-spectrum antibiotic, antifungal and antiviral regimens. PCP is treated with steroids and high-dose co-trimoxazole.

40 Pulmonary tuberculosis

Figure 40a Primary complex

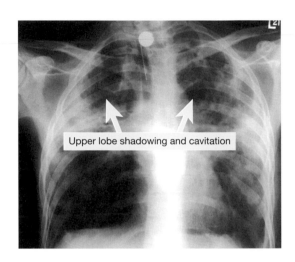

Ghon focus
and hilar
lymphadenopathy
=
'Primary complex'

Giant cells
(multinucleate)

Central caseation
('cheesy pus')

Lymphocytes

Acid-fast bacilli

Figure 40b CXR of patients with TB

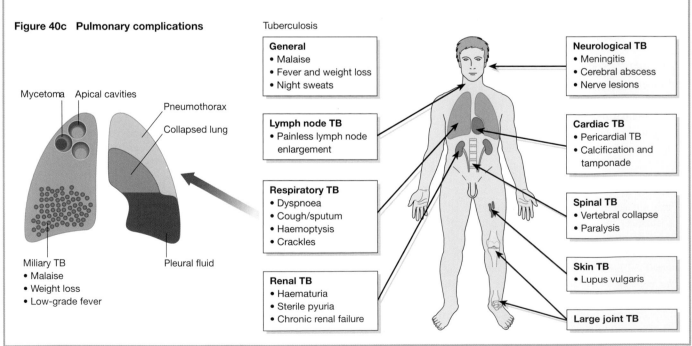

Abscess

Upper lobe shadowing and cavitation

Figure 40c Pulmonary complications

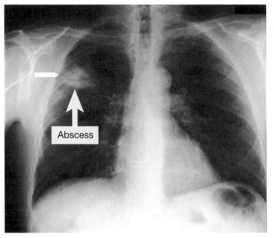

Mycetoma Apical cavities

Pneumothorax

Collapsed lung

Miliary TB
• Malaise
• Weight loss
• Low-grade fever

Pleural fluid

Tuberculosis

General
• Malaise
• Fever and weight loss
• Night sweats

Lymph node TB
• Painless lymph node
  enlargement

Respiratory TB
• Dyspnoea
• Cough/sputum
• Haemoptysis
• Crackles

Renal TB
• Haematuria
• Sterile pyuria
• Chronic renal failure

Neurological TB
• Meningitis
• Cerebral abscess
• Nerve lesions

Cardiac TB
• Pericardial TB
• Calcification and
  tamponade

Spinal TB
• Vertebral collapse
• Paralysis

Skin TB
• Lupus vulgaris

Large joint TB

The Respiratory System at a Glance, Fourth Edition. Jeremy P.T. Ward. © Jeremy P.T. Ward. Published 2015 by John Wiley & Sons, Ltd.

Worldwide, tuberculosis (TB) affects 10 million people and causes 2 million deaths each year. In developed countries it is uncommon, affecting approximately 1 per 10,000 population. Pulmonary TB is most common in Asian, Chinese and West Indian people. Airborne transmission and close contact spread the disease. Those who are elderly, malnourished or immunosuppressed (HIV infection, diabetes mellitus, corticosteroid therapy, alcoholism, intercurrent lymphoma) are more susceptible. Improved housing and nutrition reduce incidence.

Pathogenesis

Primary pulmonary TB is caused by the acid-fast bacillus *Mycobacterium tuberculosis*. The inhaled bacillus infects well-ventilated, poorly perfused upper lung lobes subpleurally. A granuloma forms (Fig. 40a) known as the Ghon focus, and with the enlarged hilar lymph node draining the affected lung is known as the 'primary complex' (Fig. 40a). This occurs over 3–8 weeks, and is accompanied by development of an inflammatory reaction to injection of tubercular protein (tuberculin) into the skin, which can be used as a diagnostic test (Mantoux or Heaf test). Complete healing usually follows, with fibrosis and calcification of the Ghon focus and immunity to further infection.

Post-primary pulmonary TB occurs if the Ghon focus fails to heal due to poor host defences, or following reactivation. It is potentially fatal. Local dissemination causes tuberculous pneumonia and pleural effusions. Bloodborne spread may affect the meninges or individual organs. In a few cases, widespread infection involves many tissues (miliary TB).

Clinical features

Primary pulmonary TB usually occurs at an early age. Often asymptomatic with no clinical signs, it may cause a mild febrile illness, erythema nodosum (painful, indurated shin lesions) and small pleural effusions. Bronchial compression by lymphadenopathy may cause wheeze and occasionally lobar collapse followed by late bronchiectasis (Chapter 36).

Post-primary TB develops over months, with malaise, anorexia, weight loss, night sweats and a productive cough. Breathlessness, chest pain, haemoptysis and cervical lymphadenopathy may occur. Clinical signs of pneumonia and pleural effusion are common, whereas lupus vulgaris (an indolent skin infection) is less frequent. Miliary TB presents with a non-specific pyrexial illness, malaise and weight loss. Sparse clinical signs include hepatomegaly and choroidal tubercles in the retina.

Investigation

Blood tests may detect anaemia, decreased sodium and increased calcium.

Mantoux test: strongly positive in post-primary pulmonary TB (>5 mm skin induration with 10 units of intradermal tuberculin; read at 3 days). Often negative in miliary TB (reduced host response) and HIV (reduced cellular immunity).

Heaf test (screening test; now less commonly used): a ring of six pinpricks is made through a tuberculin solution on the forearm. No response at 4–7 days (grade 0) demonstrates lack of immunity; 4–6 discrete nodules (grade 1) or a ring formed by coalition of all pinpricks (grade 2) indicates immunity. A single nodule formed by infilling of the ring (grade 3) represents recent contact or early tuberculous infection, and a nodule of more than 5–7 mm with surface vesicles or ulceration (grade 4) suggests infection.

Microbiology: the acid-fast bacilli may be detected in sputum or lung washings using Ziehl–Neelsen stain. However, bacilli are slow growing, and culture and drug sensitivities take 4–6 weeks. Bone marrow or cerebrospinal fluid (CSF) culture may confirm the diagnosis of miliary TB.

Histopathology: pleural aspiration with biopsy confirms TB in approximately 90% of patients with pleural effusions. Liver biopsy will isolate miliary TB in approximately 60% of cases.

Chest radiography (Fig. 40b): upper lobe shadowing is suggestive. Apical cavities, pleural effusions and pneumothoraxes may occur. In miliary TB, widespread small nodules (2–3 mm diameter) are diffusely spread throughout the lungs (miliary shadowing), and are easily missed.

Drug therapy

Prognosis is good if the patient is not immunocompromised. Good nutrition, reduced alcohol consumption and compliance with drug therapy are important factors. Uncomplicated pulmonary TB is treated for 6 months. Initially, at least three drugs are used to prevent development of resistant strains. The recommended regimen is rifampicin, pyrazinamide and isoniazid for 2 months, followed by rifampicin and isoniazid for 4 months. Additional pyridoxine prevents isoniazid-induced peripheral neuropathy. Liver function should be monitored, as rifampicin and pyrazinamide can cause liver dysfunction. If drug resistance is suspected (TB recurrence in a non-compliant patient) then a four-drug regimen (adding ethambutol) may be initiated. When culture results are available, alternative drugs replace those to which the mycobacterium is not sensitive. Ethambutol (monitor colour vision for optic neuritis), streptomycin (monitor plasma levels to avoid hearing impairment) or ciprofloxacin may be used. In severe pulmonary TB, corticosteroids occasionally improve results.

In some organs (e.g. bone), TB is treated for longer, often with additional drugs. In meningeal or cerebral TB, a four-drug regimen for 12 months with additional steroids is recommended, to ensure adequate brain penetration and to prevent cranial nerve compression by meningeal scarring.

Complications

Reactivation of old tuberculous scars may occur when a patient is immunocompromised (Fig. 40c). Chemoprophylaxis with isoniazid is often given before immunosuppressive treatment (chemotherapy, organ transplantation). Bronchiectasis and lung cavities with secondary fungal infections (mycetoma), cranial nerve lesions and renal tract obstructions may develop due to scarring associated with healing after TB. Non-compliance or inadequate treatment results in multiresistant strains of mycobacteria that may be very difficult to eradicate. Compulsory supervision and isolation of these patients may be required.

Prevention and contact tracing

Vaccination of non-immune subjects with BCG (bacillus Calmette–Guérin), a non-virulent strain of bovine TB, produces immunity and reduces the risk of pulmonary TB by 70% but is no longer routinely recommended. Community health services must be notified when a patient is diagnosed with TB, to trace contacts and prevent spread. Contacts are screened with a Mantoux test. If this suggests a risk of infection, then chest radiography and appropriate follow-up are arranged.

41 The immune-compromised patient

Figure 41a Causes of new pulmonary infiltrates

Infectious
- Bacterial pneumonia
- Fungal pneumonia (e.g. aspergillosis)
- Opportunistic pneumonia (e.g. PCP)
- Viral pneumonoia

Non-infectious
- Pulmonary oedema, ARDS
- Radiation pneumonitis
- Drug-induced, e.g. amiodarone, busulphan
- Malignant infiltration
- Pulmonary haemorrhage
- Non-specific interstitial pneumonitis

Figure 41b Infectious causes of respiratory disease in immunocompromised patients

Immunological defect	Clinical conditions	Types of infection
Neutropaenia	Chemotherapy, leukaemia, aplastic anaemia	Bacterial (e.g. *E. coli, staph aureus*) Fungal (e.g. *aspergillus*)
Impaired T-cell function	Transplantation, steroids, lymphoma, HIV infection, chemotherapy	Bacteria (e.g. mycobacteria), fungi (e.g. PCP), viruses (e.g. CMV)
Impaired B-cell function	Lymphoma, leukaemia, myeloma, hypogammaglobulinaemia	*Streptococcus pneumoniae, Haemophilus influenza*
Impaired compliment	Mannose lectin deficiency, complement deficiency	Streptococcus pneumonia

Figure 41c Clinical features of AIDS. Causes of respiratory disease and CXR infiltrates in HIV-infected patients

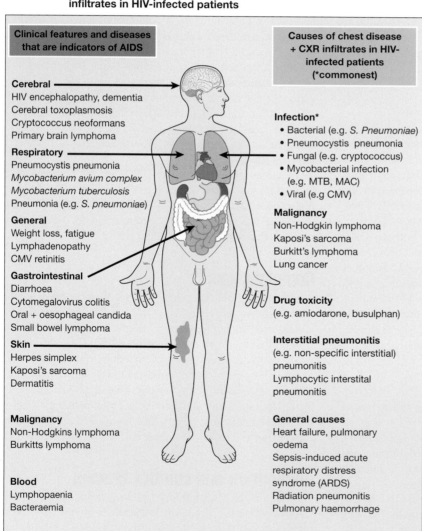

Clinical features and diseases that are indicators of AIDS

Cerebral
HIV encephalopathy, dementia
Cerebral toxoplasmosis
Cryptococcus neoformans
Primary brain lymphoma

Respiratory
Pneumocystis pneumonia
Mycobacterium avium complex
Mycobacterium tuberculosis
Pneumonia (e.g. *S. pneumoniae*)

General
Weight loss, fatigue
Lymphadenopathy
CMV retinitis

Gastrointestinal
Diarrhoea
Cytomegalovirus colitis
Oral + oesophageal candida
Small bowel lymphoma

Skin
Herpes simplex
Kaposi's sarcoma
Dermatitis

Malignancy
Non-Hodgkins lymphoma
Burkitts lymphoma

Blood
Lymphopaenia
Bacteraemia

Causes of chest disease + CXR infiltrates in HIV-infected patients (*commonest)

Infection*
- Bacterial (e.g. *S. Pneumoniae*)
- Pneumocystis pneumonia
- Fungal (e.g. cryptococcus)
- Mycobacterial infection (e.g. MTB, MAC)
- Viral (e.g CMV)

Malignancy
Non-Hodgkin lymphoma
Kaposi's sarcoma
Burkitt's lymphoma
Lung cancer

Drug toxicity
(e.g. amiodarone, busulphan)

Interstitial pneumonitis
(e.g. non-specific interstitial)
pneumonitis
Lymphocytic interstital
pneumonitis

General causes
Heart failure, pulmonary oedema
Sepsis-induced acute respiratory distress syndrome (ARDS)
Radiation pneumonitis
Pulmonary haemorrhage

Figure 41d *Pneumocystis Jirovecii* pneumonia (PCP) showing bilateral diffuse infiltrates

Figure 41e Cerebral toxoplasmosis with ring enhancement on a post-contrast CT brain scan

Mass lesion with ring enhancement

The Respiratory System at a Glance, Fourth Edition. Jeremy P.T. Ward. © Jeremy P.T. Ward. Published 2015 by John Wiley & Sons, Ltd.

The immune system is most frequently impaired after chemotherapy and in patients with human immunodeficiency virus (HIV) infection. Immunodeficiency also occurs in patients with malignancies of the lymphoproliferative system (e.g. leukaemia), immediately following bone marrow transplants (BMT) and in those on immunosuppressive drugs (e.g. steroids and azathioprine) particularly after transplant surgery (e.g. renal). Malnutrition or chronic illness (e.g. diabetes) also impairs immunity. Respiratory disease is particularly common in the immunocompromised host.

Clinical presentation is often non-specific (i.e. fever, dyspnoea, hypoxia, cough and chest discomfort) and investigation inconclusive making diagnosis difficult. In particular, pulmonary infiltrates are not always due to infection (Fig. 41a). Clinical clues include rate of onset (i.e. rapid in bacterial infection and slow with malignancy), drug therapy (e.g. methotrexate) and extrapulmonary features (e.g. Kaposi's sarcoma). Diagnostic confirmation may require invasive investigations (e.g. biopsy) with associated risks (e.g. haemorrhage).

Investigations include blood and pleural fluid microscopy, culture and serology. Sputum for *Aspergillus* or mycobacteria and 'induced' sputum for *Pneumocystis jiroveci* pneumoniae (PCP). CXR findings may be non-specific (e.g. diffuse infiltrates). Chest CT scans assess extent of lung involvement, aid invasive sampling and may be diagnostic (e.g. halo sign of aspergillosis). Early bronchoalveolar lavage (BAL) for microbiological examination, staining (e.g. fungus and virus), immunofluorescence (e.g. PCP) and serology (e.g. CMV, *Cryptococcus*) may confirm the cause (50–60%). Transbronchial, fine-needle and surgical lung biopsies have risks but also aid investigation.

Diagnosis is due to respiratory infection in >75% of cases:

- **Infection** depends on the immunological defect (Fig. 41b) and the use of prophylactic therapy (i.e. septrin to prevent PCP).
- **Non-infectious causes** present with similar clinical and CXR features to infection. They include pulmonary oedema, ARDS, malignancy (e.g. lymphoma), diffuse alveolar haemorrhage, pulmonary embolism, drug-induced disease (e.g. methotrexate), BMT-associated idiopathic pneumonia, radiation pneumonitis and chronic graft versus host disease. More than one cause is often present (30%).

Treatment is often empirical as antibiotic therapy cannot be delayed in febrile neutropenic patients, in whom infection is a medical emergency. Blood cultures should always precede antibiotics.

- **Antibiotic** choice depends on the clinical situation and local antibiotic policy. Initial treatment of immunosuppressed cases involves broad-spectrum antibiotics (±antiviral and antifungal agents). Treatment should be adjusted when results are available. PCP and CMV therapy have significant toxic side effects, but if suspicion is high, treatment is started empirically. PCP can be diagnosed for up to 2 weeks after onset of therapy. Treatment of mycobacterial infection is only started after definitive diagnosis.
- **Steroid therapy** is recommended in PCP, radiation/drug-induced pneumonitis, idiopathic pneumonia and alveolar haemorrhage.
- **Supportive therapy** includes supplemental oxygen and ventilatory support. Respiratory failure has a poor outcome in these patients.

Respiratory manifestations in the HIV-positive patient

Acquired immune deficiency syndrome (AIDS) is due to infection with HIV, which impairs and depletes CD4 T-lymphocytes (Chapter 19) (Fig. 41c). Reduction in T-lymphocyte availability predisposes to viral or fungal infections and neoplasia (Fig. 41e). Highly active antiretroviral therapy (HAART) allows T-lymphocyte population recovery, reduces susceptibility to infection and improves survival. Nevertheless, HIV patients are at increased risk of infection with common bacteria, PCP, mycobacteria and fungi.

Factors determining the type and risk of infection include the use of prophylactic antibiotics (e.g. septrin for PCP), source of infection (e.g. TB is often associated with drug abuse) and geography (e.g. histoplasmosis and coccidioidomycosis are more common in the USA). Extrapulmonary features (e.g. Kaposi's sarcoma) may suggest the cause of pulmonary disease.

1 Infectious causes

Bacterial pneumonia (e.g. *Streptococcus pneumoniae, Staphylococcus aureus, Nocardia)* is the commonest chest infection in HIV patients. Rapid onset of high fever, purulent sputum and pleuritic chest pain help distinguish bacterial pneumonia from PCP. *Legionella* infections are more common in HIV patients.

Pneumocystis jirovecii pneumonia occurs in severely immunocompromised patients (CD4 $<200 \times 10^6$/L). It has been less common since the use of septrin prophylaxis in high-risk cases. It presents with gradual onset of fever, dry cough, exertional dyspnoea, chest tightness, tachypnoea and rarely pneumothorax. Exercise-induced desaturation progresses to resting hypoxaemia. CXR shows bilateral alveolar infiltrates (Fig. 41d) but may be normal (10%) or show focal consolidation. Diagnosis requires detection of pneumocystis in induced sputum (~60–70%) or BAL (>90%). High-dose co-trimoxazole is the most effective therapy but may cause rashes (~30%), vomiting and blood disorders. Pentamidine and dapsone are second-line alternatives. High-dose steroids reduce alveolitis, respiratory failure and mortality.

Mycobacteria (e.g. *Mycobacterium tuberculosis* (MTB), *Mycobacterium avium* complex (MAC)). Globally 10% of MTB cases are also infected with HIV. However, co-infection rates vary geographically affecting 35–40% in sub-Saharan cases and 2.7% in the UK. HIV patients with previous MTB exposure have a 10% chance of reactivation, and approximately 33% of patients exposed to MTB develop primary disease. Advanced immunosuppression is typically associated with diffuse pulmonary involvement, mediastinal adenopathy and extrapulmonary involvement. Symptoms may deteriorate with the onset of HAART due to immune reconstitution. Non-tuberculous mycobacterial (NTM) infection is due to MAC in more than 90% of cases. MAC treatment is lifelong unless immune restoration is achieved with HARRT.

Viral (e.g. influenza, herpes simplex). *Cytomegalovirus* (CMV) is ubiquitous and normally harmless but can cause life-threatening pneumonia in the immunocompromised. Diagnosis requires evidence of viraemia (i.e. antigen/PCR testing on blood/BAL) or tissue invasion (e.g. 'owl eye' inclusion bodies in infected biopsy cells). Ganciclovir is the most effective antiviral agent.

Fungal (e.g. *Aspergillus*). *Cryptococcus neoformans* propagates asymptomatically in alveoli following inhalation (from bird droppings), before migrating to the CNS where it causes meningitis (±encephalitis). Onset is acute or chronic with fever, cough and non-specific CXR changes. The cryptococcal antigen test and India ink stain establish the diagnosis. Treatment is with amphotericin, flucytosine and fluconazole. In endemic areas, **histoplasmosis** and **coccidioidomycosis** may cause respiratory disease.

2 Non-infectious causes

- **Malignancies** are occasionally confused with infection in HIV patients. **Kaposi's sarcoma** is a tumour of vascular origin associated with human herpesvirus 8 infection. Clinical manifestations range from asymptomatic incidental discovery to fulminating disease, causing respiratory failure. **Non-Hodgkin's lymphoma** occurs in advanced immunosuppression and is typically aggressive B-cell or Burkitt's lymphoma, suggesting pre-existing herpesvirus infection. **Lung cancer** is also increased in HIV patients.

- **Interstitial pneumonitis** (e.g. NSIP, LIP, Chapter 32).
- **Drug-induced** lung disease or **heart failure**.

42 Lung cancer

Figure 42a Mass on CT: a >3 cm spiculated mass is seen in upper lobe of the right lung

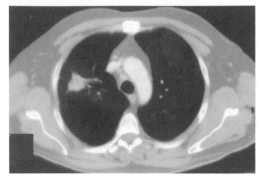

Figure 42b Fibreoptic bronchoscopy showing tumour invading bronchus

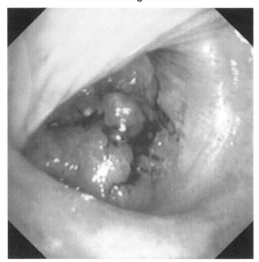

Figure 42c CXR showing squamous cell tumour in hilar region

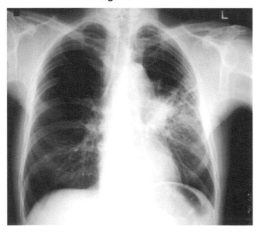

Figure 42d Staging system for non-small cell lung cancers

Stage	T (tumour)	N (node)	M (metastasis)	Key
IA	T1	N0	M0	**T1:** ≤3cm without division
IB	T2	N0	M0	**T2:** >3cm, or invasion of main bronchus >2cm from main carina, or invades visceral pleura, or bronchus causing obstruction
IIA	T1	N1	M0	
IIB	T2	N1	M0	**T3:** Invades chest wall or pleura, or main bronchus <2cm from main carina
	T3	N0	M0	**T4:** Invades adjacent structure, malignant effusion, satellite nodules
IIIA	T1, 2, 3	N2	M0	**N0:** No lymph node metastasis
	T3	N1	M0	**N1:** Ipsilateral hilar lymph nodes
IIIB	T1, 2, 3, 4	N3	M0	**N2:** Ipsilateral mediastinal or subcarinal lymph nodes
	T4	N1, 2	M0	**N3:** Contralateral, scalene or supraclavicular lymph nodes
IV	T1–4	N0–3	M1	**M0:** No distant metastasis **M1:** Any distant metastasis

Figure 42e Survival for non-small cell cancer

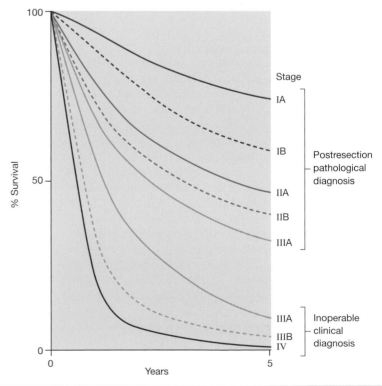

The Respiratory System at a Glance, Fourth Edition. Jeremy P.T. Ward. © Jeremy P.T. Ward. Published 2015 by John Wiley & Sons, Ltd.

More people die in the USA and Europe from **lung cancer** than from breast, prostate and colon cancer combined. Lung cancer has a **worse prognosis** than other common cancers, with an overall **5-year survival** of **13%**.

Risks

Cigarette smoking accounts for the vast majority of lung cancer cases. Risk is directly related to the duration and number of cigarettes smoked, age of initiation, depth of inhalation and levels of tar and nicotine. In heavy smokers (>20 packs/years) the lifetime risk of lung cancer is 10%, 10–30 times greater than for lifelong non-smokers (<0.3%). After quitting cigarettes, risk gradually declines over 15 years, but remains 2–5 times greater than in non-smokers. **Passive smoking** in non-smokers may increase the risk by approximately 1.5%.

Asbestos exposure is the most common occupational risk for lung cancer (Chapter 35). Tobacco smoke is synergistic with asbestosis, increasing the relative risk to 6–60 times that of a non-smoker. **Radon gas**, found naturally in rocks, soil and ground water, may also increase risk.

Classification

Lung cancers are divided pathologically into **small cell (SC,** 20–30% of total) and **non-small cell (NSC;** 70–80% of total) types. NSC types are grouped due to their similar biology, treatment and prognosis, and include **squamous cells** (30%), **large cells** (15%) and **adenocarcinoma** (33%), which are increasing in prevalence, especially in women. **Adenocarcinomas** typically present as a peripheral nodule (<3 cm) or mass (>3 cm); they are the most common type in non-smokers, and mainly arise in areas of pulmonary scarring. Bronchoalveolar cell carcinoma is an adenocarcinoma variant with low metastatic potential. **Squamous cell carcinomas** arise from the bronchial epithelium, and generally present as a central mass with tumour visible in the airway (Figs. 42a and 42b), often with symptoms due to local tumour invasion (cough, haemoptysis, chest pain and hoarseness). **Large cell carcinoma** is undifferentiated, and lacks the histological features of adenocarcinoma or squamous cell carcinoma; it generally presents as a large peripheral mass, often with metastases. **SC** carcinomas arise from neuroendocrine cells in the bronchial submucosa, and typically present as a central mass with lymph node enlargement. These are aggressive tumours that invade lymphatics and blood vessels. Nearly all have metastasized at diagnosis.

Presentation

Less than 10% of lung cancers are discovered incidentally in asymptomatic patients. Most patients are 50–70 years of age, with non-specific symptoms including new unresolving cough, haemoptysis, chest pain, hoarseness, dyspnoea on exertion, malaise and weight loss. Symptoms due to haematogenous **extrathoracic metastasis** to bone, liver, bone marrow, adrenals and brain are present in around one-third of patients at diagnosis.

Paraneoplastic syndromes – signs or symptoms associated with lung cancers that are not related directly to metastatic tumour – may precede radiographical demonstration. They may be due to secretion of hormones or hormone-like substances from tumours, or serum **autoantibodies** (e.g. anti-Hu) related to tumour antigens. SC carcinoma is associated with most paraneoplastic syndromes

including Cushing's syndrome, syndrome of inappropriate secretion of antidiuretic hormone (SIADH), Lambert–Eaton syndrome, cerebellar ataxia or idiopathic orthostatic hypotension. Squamous cell cancer may cause hypercalcaemia from release of parathyroid hormone-related peptide.

Physical findings in the lung are related to disease extent. Small **parenchymal nodules** are undetectable by physical examination. Focal findings may be due to atelectasis, airway invasion, pleural effusion (Chapter 34) or supraclavicular adenopathy. Invasion of adjacent structures may cause superior vena cava syndrome (obstruction), Horner's syndrome (autonomic overactivity) or brachial plexopathy. Digital clubbing or hypertrophic pulmonary osteoarthropathy may be present.

Evaluation

Evaluation of patients with suspected lung cancer should include demonstration of **malignancy**, **staging** and **suitability for therapy**. Radiographs provide information regarding the size and location of the tumour, benign calcification, involvement of adjacent structures, atelectasis, pleural effusion and adenopathy (Fig. 42c). **Computed tomography (CT) scans** are superior to plain X-rays. If a focal lesion does not change in 2 years, it is unlikely to be malignant. **Positron emission tomography (PET) scanning** has a high sensitivity for distinguishing benign from malignant nodules and for detecting nodal or distant metastases.

Staging is assessment of the extent of the tumour, and largely determines treatment options and prognosis. Separate staging systems are used for SC and NSC cancers. **SC cancer** is staged as either **limited** or **extensive** disease. **Limited disease** describes tumour confined to one hemithorax, including malignant pleural effusion and supraclavicular lymph node metastasis. **Extensive disease** describes metastatic spread beyond the hemithorax. SC cancer is generally an incurable disease. Standard therapy for limited disease (33%) is combination of chemotherapy and radiotherapy, with response rates approaching 90%; median survival with therapy is approximately 18 months. Standard therapy for extensive disease (66%) is chemotherapy. The response rate is approximately 70%, treatment prolonging median survival from approximately 3 months to approximately 1 year.

NSC cancer staging is based on the **tumour** (T), **node** (N) and **metastasis** (M) classification system (Fig. 42d). T3 tumours invade thoracic structures that are potentially resectable, and T4 tumours include malignant effusions or tumours invading non-resectable structures. Summation of **TNM categories** determines the stage of disease and treatment, and predicts survival (Fig. 42e). In functional patients with **stage I** or **II** disease and adequate pulmonary reserve (postoperative FEV_1>800 mL), **surgical resection** is optimal. Some patients with **stage IIIA** disease are surgical candidates. Patients with **stage IIIB** or **IV** disease are not candidates for curative resection. Unresectable disease is generally treated with **chemotherapy** and **radiation therapy**, or radiation alone. **Stage IV** disease is incurable (median survival 6–12 months). Treatment options are palliative. Painful bone metastases, brain metastasis or airway obstruction may improve with directed therapy. The benefit of aggressive chemotherapy for patients with advanced disease is modest. **Platinum-** and **taxol-based** chemotherapy regimens are currently most common for NSC cancer. Novel biological therapies include epidermal growth factor receptor blockers (e.g. **erlotinib, gefitinib**) for the 10–15% expressing the specific receptors, and protein tyrosine kinase inhibitors (e.g. **afatinib**).

43 Acute respiratory distress syndrome

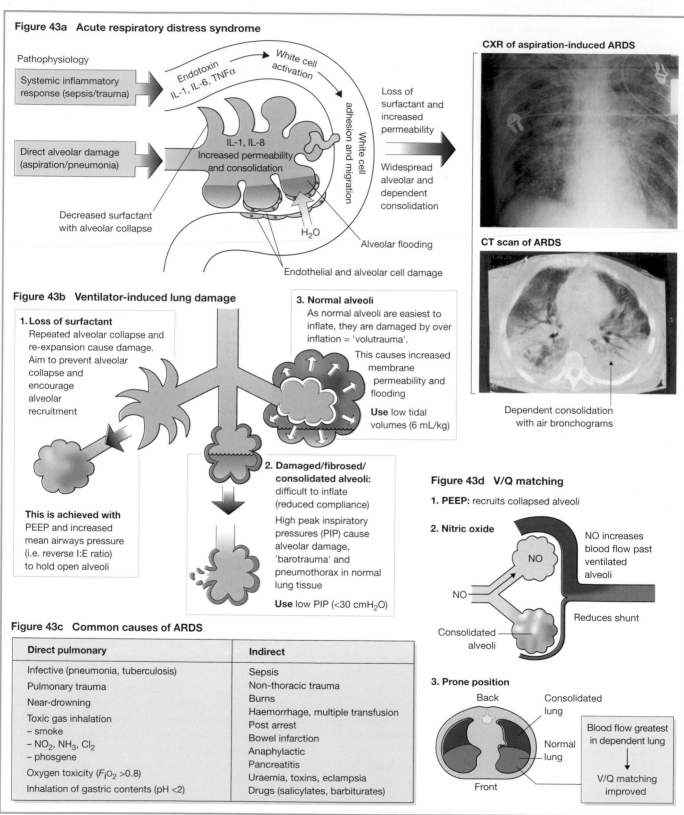

Figure 43a Acute respiratory distress syndrome

Pathophysiology

Systemic inflammatory response (sepsis/trauma)

Direct alveolar damage (aspiration/pneumonia)

Endotoxin IL-1, IL-6, TNFα

White cell activation

White cell adhesion and migration

IL-1, IL-8 Increased permeability and consolidation

Decreased surfactant with alveolar collapse

H_2O

Loss of surfactant and increased permeability

Widespread alveolar and dependent consolidation

Alveolar flooding

Endothelial and alveolar cell damage

CXR of aspiration-induced ARDS

CT scan of ARDS

Dependent consolidation with air bronchograms

Figure 43b Ventilator-induced lung damage

1. Loss of surfactant
Repeated alveolar collapse and re-expansion cause damage. Aim to prevent alveolar collapse and encourage alveolar recruitment

This is achieved with PEEP and increased mean airways pressure (i.e. reverse I:E ratio) to hold open alveoli

3. Normal alveoli
As normal alveoli are easiest to inflate, they are damaged by over inflation = 'volutrauma'.
This causes increased membrane permeability and flooding
Use low tidal volumes (6 mL/kg)

2. Damaged/fibrosed/ consolidated alveoli: difficult to inflate (reduced compliance)
High peak inspiratory pressures (PIP) cause alveolar damage, 'barotrauma' and pneumothorax in normal lung tissue
Use low PIP (<30 cmH_2O)

Figure 43d V/Q matching

1. PEEP: recruits collapsed alveoli

2. Nitric oxide
NO increases blood flow past ventilated alveoli
Reduces shunt
NO
Consolidated alveoli

3. Prone position
Back
Consolidated lung
Normal lung
Front
Blood flow greatest in dependent lung
↓
V/Q matching improved

Figure 43c Common causes of ARDS

Direct pulmonary	Indirect
Infective (pneumonia, tuberculosis)	Sepsis
Pulmonary trauma	Non-thoracic trauma
Near-drowning	Burns
Toxic gas inhalation	Haemorrhage, multiple transfusion
– smoke	Post arrest
– NO_2, NH_3, Cl_2	Bowel infarction
– phosgene	Anaphylactic
Oxygen toxicity (F_iO_2 >0.8)	Pancreatitis
Inhalation of gastric contents (pH <2)	Uraemia, toxins, eclampsia
	Drugs (salicylates, barbiturates)

The Respiratory System at a Glance, Fourth Edition. Jeremy P.T. Ward. © Jeremy P.T. Ward. Published 2015 by John Wiley & Sons, Ltd.

Acute respiratory distress syndrome (ARDS) is most simply defined as 'leaky lung syndrome' or 'low-pressure (i.e. non-cardiogenic) pulmonary oedema'. It describes an acute, diffuse inflammatory lung injury, often in previously healthy lungs (Fig. 43a) in response to a variety of direct (i.e. inhaled) or indirect (i.e. bloodborne) insults.

Diagnosis

The internationally agreed 2012 Berlin definition of ARDS requires:

- **Acute onset** within 1 week of the insult.
- **Bilateral diffuse pulmonary infiltrates** on the chest X-ray (CXR).
- **Non-cardiac origin for pulmonary oedema** (nor fluid overload).
- **Oxygenation** defines the severity of the ARDS. Mild ARDS is a P_aO_2/F_iO_2 (P/F) of 200–300 mmHg; moderate, a P/F of 100–200 mmHg and severe, a P/F of <100 mmHg (all with end expiratory pressure (PEEP)/continuous positive airways pressure (CPAP) ≥5 cmH$_2$0). P/F is calculated as follows: if P_aO_2 is 80 mmHg on 80% inspired oxygen, $P_aO_2/F_iO_2 = 80/0.8 = 100$ mmHg. Mild ARDS equates to the previous definition of acute lung injury.

Epidemiology and prognosis

The **incidence** of ARDS is approximately 2–8 cases per 100,000 population per year. Mortality is 27% in mild, 32% in moderate and ~45% in severe ARDS and is partly determined by the precipitating condition (~35% for trauma, ~50% for sepsis and ~80% for aspiration pneumonia). Age (>60 years) and sepsis are also associated with increased mortality. Early diagnosis and treatment may improve outcome. The cause of death is **multiorgan failure (MOF)**, usually due to a combination of tissue hypoxia and overwhelming secondary infection. Less than 20% of patients die from hypoxaemia alone.

Pathogenesis and causes

During the **acute inflammatory phase** of ARDS, cytokine-activated neutrophils and monocytes adhere to pulmonary endothelium or alveolar epithelium, releasing inflammatory mediators and proteolytic enzymes (Chapters 19 and 20). These damage the integrity of the alveolar–capillary membrane, increase permeability and cause alveolar oedema. Reduced surfactant production causes alveolar collapse and hyaline membrane formation. The loss of functioning alveoli and ventilation/perfusion mismatch leads to progressive hypoxaemia and respiratory failure (Figs 43a, 43b and 43c). The subsequent late **healing fibroproliferative phase** results in progressive pulmonary fibrosis and reduced compliance (stiff lungs). Associated pulmonary hypertension is partially due to activation of the coagulation cascade, with pulmonary capillary microthrombosis and regional hypoxic vasoconstriction.

Clinical features

The **acute inflammatory phase** lasts 3–10 days and results in hypoxaemia and MOF. It presents with progressive breathlessness, tachypnoea, central cyanosis, hypoxic confusion and lung crepitations. These symptoms and signs are in no way diagnostic and are shared with many other pulmonary conditions. During the later **healing, fibroproliferative phase**, pulmonary fibrosis (lung scarring) and pneumothoraxes (Chapter 37) are common. Secondary chest and systemic infections complicate both phases.

Investigations

Monitoring: Routine measurements include temperature, respiratory rate, O$_2$ saturation and urine output. In addition, the arterial and central venous pressures, the cardiac output and occasionally the left atrial pressure (using a pulmonary artery catheter) are measured **to assess fluid balance and ensure adequate tissue oxygen delivery**. Serial blood gas measurements are used to monitor gas exchange. Early detection of secondary pulmonary infection requires microbiological examination of sputum or bronchoalveolar lavage.

Radiological: Serial CXRs identify progression of **diffuse bilateral pulmonary infiltrates**. Similarly, early computed tomography (CT) scanning can identify **diffuse patchy infiltrates** with **dependent consolidation**; later scans reveal **pneumothoraxes**, **pneumatoceles** and **fibrosis**.

Management

The key to successful management of ARDS is to **establish and treat the underlying cause**. In the early stages, oxygen therapy and physiotherapy may suffice. With progressive respiratory failure, non-invasive ventilation – with CPAP or non-invasive positive pressure ventilation (NIPPV) – or full mechanical ventilation and high-inspired oxygen concentrations may be required to maintain adequate ventilation and oxygenation. The high airway pressures needed to achieve normal tidal volumes during mechanical ventilation often result in lung damage (barotrauma), including pneumothorax and lung cysts. This ventilator-induced lung injury and oxygen toxicity ($F_iO_2 > 0.8$) must be prevented, as these contribute to mortality and MOF (Fig. 43b).

The basic principles of mechanical ventilation are to **limit pressure-induced damage, optimize oxygenation** and **avoid circulatory compromise** (reduced cardiac output and blood pressure due to high intrathoracic pressures; see also Chapter 44). A 'protective lung ventilation strategy' of low tidal volumes (6 mL/kg) and low peak inspiratory pressures (<30 cmH$_2$O) reduces lung damage, complications and mortality. **Alveolar recruitment** (of collapsed alveoli) is achieved with high positive end-expiratory pressures (PEEP >10 cmH$_2$O) or long inspiratory–expiratory (I:E) times. The CO$_2$ retention ('permissive hypercapnia') resulting from this strategy of low tidal volume ventilation can be tolerated for long periods.

Conservative (i.e. 'dry') fluid management limits alveolar oedema related to increased alveolar permeability. The aim must be to maintain adequate perfusion of other organs while using the lowest possible left atrial pressures. In the acute situation, diuretics may be essential to correct hypoxaemia by reducing extravascular lung water. Thereafter, combinations of systemic vasodilators (after load reduction of the left heart), inotropes and vasoconstrictor agents may be used to achieve adequate cardiac output and perfusion pressures at low left atrial filling pressures.

Essential general measures include good nursing care, physiotherapy, nutrition and infection control. Reducing fever (shivering) and controlling anxiety with sedation decrease metabolic demand. **No drug therapy has been consistently beneficial** in early ARDS, including steroids, anti-inflammatory agents, anticytokines or surfactant therapy. However, 7–10 days after onset, steroid therapy may prevent the development of subsequent pulmonary fibrosis. **Inhaled nitric oxide** and nursing the patient in the **prone position** improve gas exchange by increasing perfusion to ventilated areas of lung, but no survival benefit has been demonstrated (Fig. 43d). **Extracorporeal membrane oxygenation (ECMO)** techniques to oxygenate blood or remove CO$_2$ are effective in children, and increasing evidence suggests benefit in adults.

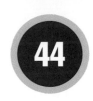

44 Mechanical ventilation

Figure 44a Indications for mechanical ventilation or support in adults

Surgery General anaesthesia with neuromuscular blockade Postoperative management following major surgery	**Cervical cord damage above C4** Neck fractures
Respiratory centre depression Usually when P_aCO_2 >7–8kPa (50–60mmHg) Head injury Drug overdose, e.g. opiates, barbiturates Raised intracranial pressure: cerebral haemorrhage/ tumours/meningitis/encephalitis Status epilepticus	**Neuromuscular disorders** – when VC <20–30mL/kg Guillain–Barré Myasthenia gravis Poliomyelitis Polyneuritis
	Chest wall disorders Kyphoscoliosis Trauma: especially flail segment (multiple rib fractures → section of chest wall unattached)
Lung disease Pneumonia Acute respiratory distress syndrome (ARDS) Severe asthma attack Acute exacerbation of chronic obstructive pulmonary disease (COPD), cystic fibrosis Trauma–lung contusion Pulmonary oedema	**Other** Cardiac arrest Severe circulatory shock Resistant hypoxia in type 1 respiratory failure (reduces oxygen consumption)

Figure 44b Nasal mask and NIPPV

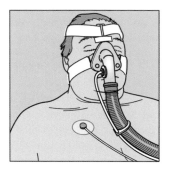

Figure 44c Airway pressure profiles in different types of ventilation

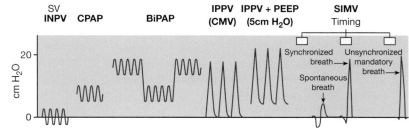

SV = spontaneous ventilation, **INPV** = intermittent negative pressure ventilation, **CPAP** = continuous positive airway pressure, **BiPAP** = biphasic continuous airway pressure (trace shown is fixed time period BiPAP), **IPPV** = intermittent positive pressure ventilation (= CMV), **CMV** = controlled mechanical ventilation, **PEEP** = positive end-expiratory pressure, **SIMV** = synchronized intermittent mandatory ventilation. If a spontaneous breath occurs in the timing window it triggers a synchronized ventilator breath and if not a mandatory breath is given soon after the timing window.

Figure 44d Complications of mechanical ventilation

Risks during endotracheal intubation or tracheostomy Myocardial depression from anaesthetic Aspiration of gastric contents Fall in P_aCO_2 during apnoea Reflex bronchoconstriction, laryngospasm and bradycardia	**Risks associated with sedation and paralysis** Cardiac depression Depression of respiratory drive (delays weaning) Increases danger of disconnection/ventilator failure
Risks of endotracheal intubation and tracheostomy Intubation of the oesophagus Intubation of a bronchus Blockage/accidental extubation Laryngeal/tracheal damage or stenosis Infection	**Risks associated with mechanical ventilation** High airway pressure →barotrauma Alveolar overdistension →volutrauma: • Pneumothorax, pneumomediastinum • Subcutaneous emphysema (= air in skin) • Structural damage to lung, airways and capillaries • Bronchopulmonary dysplasia (see Chapter 18)
Risks associated with high inspired oxygen (see Chapter 45)	

Mechanical ventilation is usually used to prevent or treat type 2 respiratory (ventilatory) failure. The main indications in adults are listed in Figure 44a.

Types of mechanical ventilation

Inspiratory muscle paralysis by poliomyelitis was a common reason for mechanical ventilation in the first half of the 20th century (Fig. 44c). It was usually performed by **intermittent negative pressure ventilation (INPV)**, which is still occasionally used today. Patients are placed inside a **tank ventilator** sealed at the neck, and tank pressure is intermittently lowered, expanding the chest and lowering intrapleural pressure as in spontaneous breathing. Disadvantages of this **iron lung** include claustrophobia, discomfort, difficult nursing care and the bulk and expense of the equipment. **Jacket** and **cuirass ventilators** produce a negative pressure just around the chest, but difficulty in achieving a satisfactory seal limits their use to patients only needing ventilatory augmentation.

From the 1950s, **intermittent positive pressure ventilation (IPPV; controlled mechanical ventilation, CMV)** quickly replaced INPV for most purposes. Air is driven into the lungs by raising airway pressure, usually via an endotracheal or tracheostomy tube. Expiration is achieved by allowing pressure to fall to zero. This simple form of IPPV is used during routine surgery. Typical initial adult settings for IPPV are:

Tidal volume, $V_T = 8–12$ mL/kg
Respiratory frequency, $f = 8–14$ breaths/min
Minute ventilation, $V(= V_T \times f) \approx 6000$ mL/min
Inspiratory time/expiratory time = 1:2–1:3

Minute ventilation is adjusted to maintain P_aCO_2 at about 5 kPa (37 mmHg). A slightly lower P_aCO_2 may be used initially in the presence of raised intracranial pressure. Accepting a higher P_aCO_2 (**permissive hypercapnia**) may prevent the need for excessively high airway pressures. P_aO_2 is maintained above 10 kPa (75 mmHg) by adjusting inspired FO_2. The lowest concentration needed is used, usually in the range 30–60%. It may be preferable to accept a slightly lower PO_2 than to use more than 60% for long periods.

Microprocessor control of ventilators has permitted development of numerous variations of IPPV. For example, in non-paralysed patients, the positive pressure may be synchronized with spontaneous breaths and a mandatory breath given if no spontaneous breaths occur in a preset time (**synchronized intermittent mandatory ventilation, SIMV**). In another form, the ventilator operates only where spontaneous ventilation falls below a preset minimum (**mandatory minute ventilation, MMV**).

If, instead of allowing airway pressure to fall to zero, a small positive pressure is maintained throughout expiration (**positive end-expiratory pressure, PEEP**), there is a reduction in V_A/Q mismatching and an improvement in P_aO_2 in some conditions, such as acute respiratory distress syndrome (ARDS). This occurs because PEEP increases functional residual capacity (FRC) and reduces the closure of airways and alveoli towards the end of expiration. Unfortunately, intrathoracic pressure is raised, impairing venous return, and occasionally the fall in cardiac output can reduce tissue oxygen delivery despite the increased P_aO_2.

The increased mean airway pressure caused by PEEP also increases the risk of barotrauma. A good compromise is to use the minimum PEEP required to keep PO_2 at an acceptable level (>8 kPa, 60 mmHg) when breathing 50–60% oxygen.

Non-invasive respiratory support

Non-invasive ventilation avoids the use of tracheal intubation or tracheostomy. An example is INPV (above), but this is no longer widely used. In contrast, non-invasive positive pressure techniques using either a nasal mask (Fig. 44b) or sometimes a full face mask are increasingly being used.

In **continuous positive airway pressure (CPAP)**, a standing pressure of 5–10 cmH$_2$O is applied to a nasal or face mask in a spontaneously breathing patient (Fig. 44c). This has several potential beneficial effects. First, it helps prevent upper airway collapse in **obstructive sleep apnoea**. In interstitial diseases such as **ARDS**, it recruits alveoli, reducing V_A/Q mismatching. FRC is increased, and this may increase lung compliance by moving the patient onto the steep part of the pressure–volume curve (Chapter 6). CO$_2$ retention may be a problem during CPAP, which may be improved by using biphasic or bilevel positive pressure ventilation (BiPAP). BiPAP alternates between high and low pressure either for fixed time periods (Fig. 44c) or between inspiration and expiration, making expiration easier and improving the emptying of the lungs.

CPAP may improve oxygenation and may aid the patient's own respiratory efforts, but it cannot produce ventilation by itself. In contrast, **non-invasive intermittent positive pressure ventilation (NIPPV)** is IPPV delivered by face or, more usually, nasal mask. For it to be used successfully, the patient must be cooperative and introduced to the technique gradually, to allow synchronization of his or her breathing with the ventilator. Its use includes nocturnal ventilation of patients with chronic respiratory failure due to neuromuscular disease or thoracic deformity. It is well established for the treatment of respiratory failure caused by acute exacerbations of chronic obstructive pulmonary disease (COPD), avoiding the need for intubation and improving survival. It is increasingly being used for a range of other conditions as an alternative to standard IPPV.

In summary, the main beneficial effect of **CPAP** is recruitment of alveoli. The reduction in collapse sometimes also gives rise to a reduction in the work of breathing. In contrast, **NIPPV** is used to reduce or take over the work of breathing rather than to recruit alveoli. This may be of benefit in the tired (e.g. COPD) patient.

Weaning the patient off the ventilator following surgery is usually achieved by reversing neuromuscular blockade and lightening the anaesthetic level. With Intensive Care Unit patients, weaning may be more difficult. Several techniques are used, including removing mechanical ventilation for progressively longer periods, or by using a spontaneous breathing mode (e.g. SIMV), and pressure support in which support is progressively reduced. CPAP applied via the endotracheal tube may also help the weaning process.

Problems are hard to predict accurately, but are most likely following prolonged ventilation, in debilitated patients, or in those with neuromuscular or chronic respiratory disease. A pattern of rapid shallow breathing 5 minutes after disconnection from the ventilator is one of the more useful predictors of failure.

Complications of mechanical ventilation are numerous, and are listed in Figure 44d.

45 Oxygenation and oxygen therapy

Figure 45a Indications for acute oxygen therapy

1. Cardiac and respiratory arrest

2. Hypoxaemia (P_aO_2 <8kPa, S_aO_2 <90%)

3. Hypotension (systolic BP <90 mmHg)

4. Low cardiac output

5. CO poisoning

6. Respiratory distress (respiratory rate >24/min)
   if oxygenation in doubt

Figure 45b Risks associated with high-dose oxygen therapy

1. **Carbon dioxide retention:**
   ~10% of breathless patients, mainly COPD, have type 2 respiratory failure (RF).
   ~40–50% of COPD patients are at risk of type 2 RF

2. **Rebound hypoxaemia:**
   occurs if oxygen is suddenly withdrawn in type 2 RF

3. **Absorption collapse**
   O_2 in poorly ventilated alveoli is rapidly absorbed whereas N_2 absorption is slow,
   so high FO_2 can cause collapse

4. **Pulmonary oxygen toxicity**
   F_iO_2>60% may damage alveolar membranes causing ARDS if inhaled for
   >24–48 hrs (Chapter 41). Hyperoxia can cause coronary and cerebral vasospasm

5. **Fire**
   Deaths and burns occur in smokers during O_2 therapy

6. **Paul–Bert effect**
   Hyperbaric O_2 can cause cerebral vasoconstriction and epileptic fits

Figure 45c Oxygen delivery devices

1. Variable performance devices

Air is entrained during breathing whilst oxygen is delivered from a reservoir (i.e. mask, reservoir bag, nasopharynx)

The F_iO_2 delivered to the lungs depends on the oxygen flow rate, the patient's inspiratory flow, respiratory rate and the amount of air entrained

e.g. Figure (i) 'Low-flow face masks', O_2 flows at ~2–10 L/min into the mask and is supplemented by air drawn into the mask. The F_iO_2 achieved depends on ventilation

Ventilation = 5 L/min
O2 flow = 2 L/min; air (21% O_2) flow = 3 L/min
F_iO_2 = (2+0.21 x 3)/5 x 100 = **53%**

Ventilation = 25 L/min
O_2 flow = 2 L/min; air (21% O_2) flow = 23 L/min
F_iO_2 = (2+0.21 x 23)/25 x 100 = **27%**

These devices cannot be used if accurate control of F_iO_2 is desirable, e.g. COPD with hypercapnia

Examples of variable performance devices are 'low-flow' facemasks (see i), nasal cannulae (see ii) and non-rebreathing face masks with reservoir bags (see iii)

(i) 'Low-flow' facemask

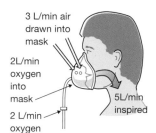

3 L/min air drawn into mask

2L/min oxygen into mask

2 L/min oxygen

5L/min inspired

F_iO_2 can be 60% at 15 L/min O_2

O_2 flows at ~2–15 L/min into the mask and is supplemented by air drawn into the mask. Flow rate must be > 5 L/min to prevent CO_2 rebreathing

(ii) Nasal cannulae

O_2 flow rates up to 4 L/min. Higher rates dry mucosa

F_iO_2 is between 24 and 35%

The O_2 flow is constant so F_iO_2 varies with ventilatory volume. More comfortable and not removed during eating or coughing.
O_2 inhaled even when mouth breathing

(iii) Non-rebreathing and anaesthetic masks

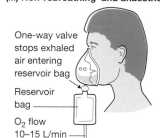

One-way valve stops exhaled air entering reservoir bag

Reservoir bag

O_2 flow 10–15 L/min

F_iO_2 is 60–100% at O_2 flow rates of 10–15 L/min

High (10–15 L/min) flow rates of O_2 provide high F_iO_2 > 60% and up to 100%

Non-rebreathing masks have a reservoir bag which should be filled before use. They increase F_iO_2 by preventing O_2 loss during expiration

2. Fixed performance devices

Are independent of the patient's pattern of breathing and inspiratory volume

Figure (iv) illustrates that a fixed O_2 flow through a Venturi valve entrains the correct proportion of air to achieve the required O_2 concentration

This system delivers more gas than is inspired (i.e. >30 L/min). Consequently, F_iO_2 is less affected by the breathing pattern. The resulting masks are high flow, low concentration and fixed performance

Used in patients with COPD and respiratory failure to avoid CO_2 retention

(iv) 'High-flow' (Venturi), low concentration face mask

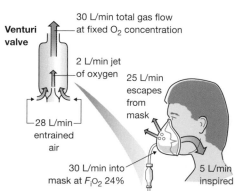

Venturi valve

30 L/min total gas flow at fixed O_2 concentration

2 L/min jet of oxygen

25 L/min escapes from mask

28 L/min entrained air

30 L/min into mask at F_iO_2 24%

5 L/min inspired

Venturi valves are colour coded and deliver 24, 28, 31, 35, 40 or 60% F_iO_2 for a fixed flow rate

Continuous positive airways pressure (CPAP) masks
Use a tight fitting mask and a flow generator to deliver a fixed F_iO_2 with a positive pressure (5–10 cm/H_2O) throughout the respiratory cycle

Sufficient O_2 must be delivered to the tissues to support metabolism, and the tissues must be able to utilize it. **Tissue hypoxia** can be caused by **low arterial** P_{O_2} and therefore **blood O_2 content** (hypoxaemia); inadequate **tissue blood flow** (ischaemia, cardiac failure, emboli); low **haemoglobin concentration** (anaemia); abnormal **oxygen dissociation curve** (haemoglobinopathies, CO poisoning); and **poisoning of intracellular oxygen usage** (e.g. cyanide and sepsis). Tissue hypoxia occurs within 4 minutes of failure of any of these systems because tissue and lung O_2 reserves are small. Clinical features are often non-specific, including altered mental state, dyspnoea, hyperventilation, arrhythmias and hypotension (see Chapter 25). Anaemia and abnormal dissociation curves are discussed in Chapter 8.

Measuring tissue hypoxia

Arterial oxygen saturation (S_aO_2) is measured with a **pulse oximeter**, and partial pressure of oxygen (P_aO_2) by **blood gas analysis**. S_aO_2 should be measured regularly in all breathless patients. However, both P_aO_2 and S_aO_2 can be normal when tissue hypoxia is caused by low cardiac output states, anaemia and failure of tissue O_2 use. In these circumstances, **mixed venous oxygen partial pressure** (P_v–O_2), which is measured in blood taken from a pulmonary artery catheter, approximates to mean tissue P_{O_2}. However, severe hypoxia in a single organ (e.g. due to an arterial embolus) may be associated with a normal P_aO_2, S_aO_2 and P_vO_2.

Oxygen therapy

Given correctly O_2 is a lifesaving drug, but it is often used without appropriate evaluation of potential benefits and side effects. Figure 45a lists indications for initiating O_2 therapy, whereas Figure 45b lists potential risks. Immediate assessment of airways, breathing and circulation is essential to confirm airway patency and good circulation. Figure 45c illustrates important features of O_2 delivery systems. The aims of O_2 therapy depend on the risk of developing **type 2 (hypercapnic, CO_2 retaining) respiratory failure** (Chapter 25):

- **In normal patients** (low risk of type 2 respiratory failure) aim for an S_aO_2 of 94–98% (92–98% if >70 years), that is, the plateau of the O_2–haemoglobin dissociation curve; increasing P_aO_2 further has no impact on O_2 delivery as little O_2 is dissolved in plasma (Chapter 8).
- **In patients at risk of type 2 respiratory failure** (e.g. COPD) target S_aO_2 should be 88–92% pending arterial blood gas (ABG) analysis. A higher S_aO_2 has few advantages but may result in hypoventilation, hypercapnia and respiratory acidosis in patients dependent on hypoxic respiratory drive (Chapter 12).

Initial O_2 dose and delivery method depends on cause of hypoxia:

- **High-dose supplemental oxygen (>60%)** is delivered through a non-rebreathing, reservoir mask at 10–15 L/min (Fig. 45c(iii)). Indicating conditions include cardiac or respiratory arrest, shock, major trauma, sepsis, CO poisoning and critical illness. Once the patient is stable, the O_2 dose is reduced to maintain an S_aO_2 of 92–98%. Seriously ill patients at risk of hypercapnic respiratory failure (HCRF) are initially treated with high-dose O_2 pending ABG analysis.

- **Moderate-dose supplemental oxygen (40–60%)** is given in serious illnesses (e.g. pneumonia) through nasal cannulae (2–6 L/min) or simple face masks (5–10 L/min), aiming for an S_aO_2 of 92–98% (Figs. 45c(i) and 45c(ii)). A reservoir mask is substituted if this is not achieved.
- **Low-dose (controlled) supplemental oxygen (24–28%)** is delivered through a fixed performance Venturi mask (Fig. 45c(iv)). It is indicated in patients at risk of **CO_2-retaining, type 2 respiratory failure**, including COPD, neuromuscular disease, chest wall disorders and cystic fibrosis. Target S_aO_2 is 88–92% whilst awaiting ABG results. If P_aCO_2 is normal, the S_aO_2 is adjusted to 92–98% (except in patients with previous type 2 respiratory failure) and ABG rechecked at 1 hour. A raised P_aCO_2 and bicarbonate with normal pH suggest longstanding hypercapnia and type 2 respiratory failure (Chapter 11); the target S_aO_2 should therefore be 88–92% with repeat ABG at 1 hour. If the patient is hypercapnic (P_aCO_2>6 kPa) and acidotic (pH <7.35), non-invasive ventilation (NIV, Chapter 44) should be considered. Venturi masks are replaced with nasal cannulae (1–2 L/min) when the patient is stable. An O_2 alert card and Venturi mask are issued to patients with previous type 2 respiratory failure to warn future emergency staff of the potential risk.

Oxygen therapy is of little benefit in 'normoxic' patients because the haemoglobin is fully saturated. Restoration of tissue blood flow is often more important in these cases. In myocardial infarction, drug overdoses, metabolic disorders, hyperventilation or during labour in non-hypoxic pregnant women, O_2 therapy is of little value. It may actually be harmful in normoxic patients with strokes, paraquat poisoning or acid inhalation, and to the fetus in normoxic obstetric emergencies. However, in **CO poisoning** high-dose O_2 is essential, despite a normal P_aO_2, to reduce the half-life of carboxyhaemoglobin (Chapter 8).

Stop oxygen therapy when the patient is clinically stable on low-dose O_2 (e.g. 1–2 L/min) and S_aO_2 is within the desired range on two consecutive occasions. Monitor S_aO_2 for 5 minutes after stopping O_2 and recheck at 1 hour.

Other techniques to improve oxygenation

1 Anaemia: Failure of tissue O_2 delivery is best corrected by raising haemoglobin concentration e.g. by blood transfusion.
2 Block of airways by mucus and retention of secretions (e.g. cystic fibrosis, Chapter 36) requires physiotherapy, mucolytic agents and occasionally bronchoscopy to remove blockages and improve alveolar ventilation.
3 Fluid restriction reduces alveolar oedema when alveolar permeability is increased (e.g. ARDS, Chapter 43).
4 Alveolar recruitment improves oxygenation by reducing V_A/Q mismatch and shunt (Chapters 14 and 15). Simple postural changes may improve oxygenation. Sitting upright optimizes V_A/Q matching in the alert patient. Regular turning and prone positioning improve secretion drainage and oxygenation in supine patients. Techniques that increase mean alveolar pressures (e.g. PEEP, CPAP and increased inspiratory/expiratory ratio) also improve alveolar recruitment and oxygenation (Chapter 44).
5 Ventilatory support (e.g. NIV) improves oxygenation by correcting hypoventilation and associated hypercapnia (Chapters 9 and 44).

46 Sleep apnoea

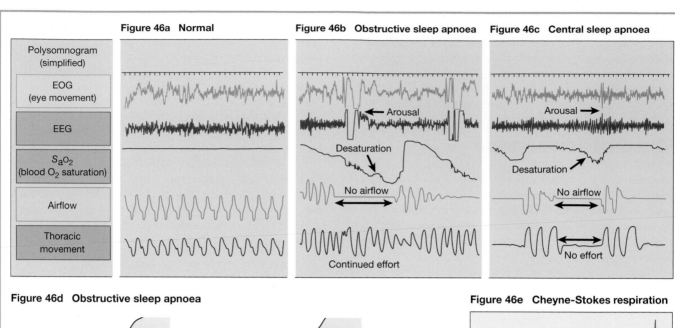

Figure 46a Normal

Figure 46b Obstructive sleep apnoea

Figure 46c Central sleep apnoea

Polysomnogram (simplified)

EOG (eye movement)

EEG

S_aO_2 (blood O_2 saturation)

Airflow

Thoracic movement

Arousal

Desaturation

No airflow

Continued effort

Arousal

Desaturation

No airflow

No effort

Figure 46d Obstructive sleep apnoea

Tongue

Uvula

Blocked airway

Pharynx

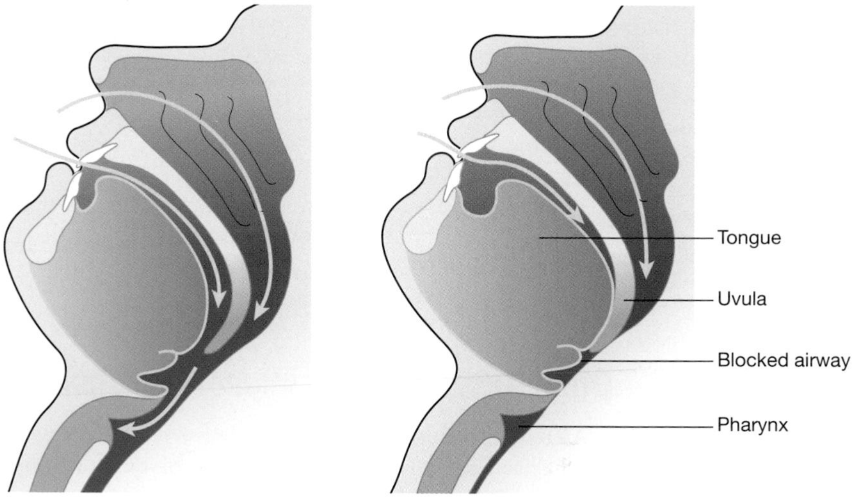

Normal airflow

Obstructed airflow

Figure 46e Cheyne-Stokes respiration

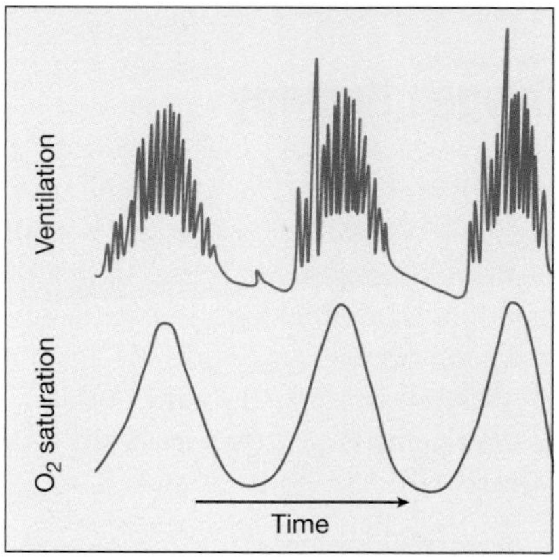

Ventilation

O_2 saturation

Time

Cheyne-Stokes respiration occurs in heart failure and at altitude, and is characterized by slowly increasing and decreasing depth of each breath

The Respiratory System at a Glance, Fourth Edition. Jeremy P.T. Ward. © Jeremy P.T. Ward. Published 2015 by John Wiley & Sons, Ltd.

Sleep apnoea (or sleep-disordered breathing) is common, with a vast potential for improvement in quality of life. It is caused by obstruction of the upper airways (**obstructive sleep apnoea; OSA**), and more rarely **central sleep apnoea (CSA)**, where the central control of ventilation is disturbed. It can lead to significant sleep deprivation and fragmentation and thus daytime hypersomnolence (sleepiness), with consequent decreased quality of life, mental and physical performance, and increased risk of accidents and cardiovascular disease, such as hypertension. Sleep-disordered breathing is diagnosed using **polysomnography** (Fig. 46a), which records the electroencephalography (EEG) for sleep patterns, movements of abdomen and thorax to assess breathing, oronasal flow and oximetry for O_2 saturation. Normal sleep (Fig. 46a) consists of rapid eye movement (**REM**; ~25%) and non-rapid eye movement (**NREM**) sleep. REM sleep is characterized by an awake-pattern EEG, voluntary muscle atonia and dreaming. Ventilatory drive is normally diminished in REM sleep, causing a slight fall in P_aO_2 and a rise in P_aCO_2. Sleep apnoea is associated with multiple periods of hypoxaemia and partial awakenings (Figs. 46 and 46c).

Obstructive sleep apnoea

OSA is characterized by absence of airflow with continued respiratory effort (Fig. 46b). About 90% of patients with sleep apnoea have OSA. OSA is far more common in males than females, and is associated with alcohol consumption, increasing age, obesity, increased neck circumference, hypertension and hypothyroidism. Obstruction typically occurs in the upper airway and pharynx, and is related to the normal decrease in upper airway muscle tone that occurs in REM sleep coupled with narrowing of the pharyngeal airways due to obesity or enlarged tonsils. Neuromuscular disease (e.g. stroke) and muscle relaxants (e.g. alcohol and sedatives) may further reduce upper airway muscle tone. These factors, in conjunction with individual anatomy and posture, result in airway obstruction during inspiration, when airway pressure is reduced (Fig. 46d).

Apnoea resolves with arousal and restoration of muscle tone. Although hundreds or thousands of episodes of apnoea and arousal may occur each night in severe cases, patients are often unaware of them; sleep partners commonly report **loud snoring**, snorting or apnoea. Patients commonly report unrefreshing sleep and nocturia, develop **daytime hypersomnolence** and **gain weight**, and may show pedal oedema, nasal congestion, enlarged tongue, shallow palate, enlarged uvula or retrognathia. Most patients have normal arterial daytime blood gases and haemoglobin. In chronic obstructive pulmonary disease (COPD), **nocturnal hypoxia** can be severe even with mild OSA, as gas exchange is already compromised.

Polysomnography reveals repeated episodes of OSA or hypopnoea (reduced airflow with oxygen desaturation or arousal), which terminate with arousal (Fig. 46b). These episodes are quantified by the **apnoea plus hypopnoea index** (AHI, episodes/hour). Normal sleep has an AHI of less than 10. Severe OSA usually has an AHI of more than 40. Obstructive episodes can cause **pulmonary hypertension** (Chapter 29) from hypoxic pulmonary vasoconstriction. Systemic blood pressure increases during apnoea, possibly due to sympathetic stimulation, and left ventricle (LV) afterload increases during obstructive apnoeas due to the marked fall in pleural pressure.

There is a strong association between OSA and systemic hypertension, and cardiovascular risk is sharply increased. OSA is thought to promote atherosclerosis, defective cardiovascular regulation and impaired sensitivity of the arterial chemoreceptors; it is known to impair cognitive function. The cause is unknown, but may be related to increased oxidant stress caused by intermittent hypoxia.

Morbidly obese patients with severe OSA may develop **obesity hypoventilation syndrome** (OHS, Pickwick syndrome). OHS is associated with daytime hypoventilation (P_aCO_2 >45 mmHg), and prevalence increases sharply with BMI. Multiple factors contribute to OHS, including depressed chemoreceptor function and respiratory control.

Management of OSA requires relief of obstruction. Moderate weight loss (≥10%) often results in substantial improvements, as does limiting evening consumption of alcohol. When OSA is significant, **nasal continuous positive airway pressure** (CPAP, Chapter 44) is the most commonly prescribed therapy, but 50% of patients do not comply in the long term. Some patients respond to oral appliances or removal of tonsils, though uvulopalatopharyngoplasty (surgery) is rarely beneficial. O_2 alone may decrease or eliminate hypoxia, but not the obstruction or arousals.

Central sleep apnoea

CSA is characterized by cessation of airflow during sleep without evidence of respiratory effort, and is due to a **loss or inhibition of central respiratory drive** (Fig. 46). Patients with CSA may be subdivided into those with daytime hypercapnia or normocapnia. CSA with daytime hypercapnia is usually due to central alveolar hypoventilation, neuromuscular disease or restrictive chest wall disease (e.g. kyphoscoliosis). Central alveolar hypoventilation may be congenital or due to brainstem disease and strokes (see also Ondine's curse; Chapter 13). Neuromuscular causes include muscular dystrophy, phrenic nerve dysfunction, myositis (muscle inflammation) and myasthenia gravis. Inspiratory muscle impairment in restrictive or obstructive (e.g. COPD) respiratory disease can lead to increased use of accessory muscles during ventilation, but voluntary muscle atonia during REM sleep can therefore lead to profound hypoxaemia.

Cheyne–Stokes respiration is an abnormal pattern of breathing characterized by gradual waxing and waning of the depth of breathing, leading to periods of hypoventilation and desaturation (Fig. 46d). It is commonly experienced in patients with heart failure and at altitude. The underlying causes are not fully understood, but may include dysregulation of feedback from the chemoreceptors (Chapter 12). Under these conditions hypoxaemia can lead to hyperventilation and thus hypocapnia and alkalosis. On sleeping, ventilatory drive may be depressed, leading to hypercapnia or apnoea and hypoxaemia, which causes arousal and hyperventilation again, and the sequence repeats throughout the sleeping period.

Therapy for CSA depends on symptoms. Patients with a CNS cause for hypoventilation ('won't breathe') may benefit from a respiratory stimulant. Patients with weakness or chest wall disease ('can't breathe') benefit from assisted mechanical ventilation, specifically non-invasive intermittent positive pressure ventilation (**NIPPV**, Chapter 44). Cheyne–Stokes respiration can be improved by treatment of the underlying condition (heart failure) or raising the inspired O_2.

Index

abdominal
  breathing 5
  muscles 5
accessory inspiratory muscles 5
acclimatization 25, 33
acidaemia 23
acid–base
  balance 20–21
  disorders 22–3
acidosis 21, 23
  hyperchloraemic 23
  metabolic 23, 25
acids
  strong 21
  weak 21
acrolein 74
acute mountain sickness 33
acute respiratory distress syndrome
  (ARDS) 75, 90–91
acute respiratory failure 23, 55
adaptive immune
  mechanisms 41
adenocarcinomas 89
adrenaline (epinephrine) 15
afatinib 89
AIDS 86–7
air trapping 15
airways 3
  narrowing 57
  resistance 13–15, 47
  wall remodelling 57
albuterol 58
alcohol use/abuse 45
aldehydes 74
alkalaemia 23
alkalosis 21, 23
  metabolic 23, 25
allelic exclusion 41
allergic asthma 57
allergy 41
alpha1-antitrypsin 39
  deficiency 36, 39, 61
altitude acclimatization 25, 33
altitude, breathing at 9, 25, 32–3
alveoli 38
  alveolar air equation 30–31
  alveolar–capillary membrane 3,
    10–11, 35, 47, 54–5, 91
  dead space 3
  ducts and sacs 2–3, 38
  epithelium 10–11
  gas 3
  interdependence 13
  lining fluid 13

pressure 6–7
ventilation 3
ambient temperature and pressure
  saturated with water (ATPS) 9
aminophylline 58–9
ammonia 74
anaemia 16–17, 95
anaerobic
  pneumonia 81
  threshold 33
anatomical dead space 3
angle
  of Louis 2, 5
  of rib 5
anion gap 22–3
antibodies 40
anticholinergics 61
anticoagulation 63
antidepressants 53
antigen-presenting cells (APCs) 39–41,
  57
antigens 41, 57
anti-inflammatory cytokines 39
anti-neutrophil cytoplasmic antibodies
  (ANCA) 67
anti-proteases 39
aorta 24
aortic bodies 24–5
apneusis 27
apneustic centre 27
apnoea 27
arterial
  blood gases 47
  hypoxia 54
  oxygen saturation 47
asbestos 75
  and lung cancer 89
  bodies 75
asbestosis 75
aspiration pneumonia 81
asthma 44, 55, 75
  pathophysiology 56–7
  treatment 58–9
  uncontrolled 59
atelectasis 13, 29
atopic asthma 57
auscultation 44–5
autoregulation 29
autosomal recessive trait 77

B cell receptors (BCRs) 41
bagassosis 74
barometric pressure 8
barrel chest 7, 61

base excess 23
beclomethasone 59
bellows spirometer 7
bends, the 33
β2-agonists 58–9, 61
bicarbonate anions 19, 21
birth 34–5
blood–brain barrier 25
blue asbestos 75
blue bloater 55
body plethysmography 7, 46–7
body temperature and pressure saturated
  with water (BTPS) 9
Bohr effect 17
Bohr equation for dead space
  measurement 2–3
Bohr shift 17
bone morphogenetic protein receptor type
  2 (BMPR2) 63
Bötzinger complex 26–7
Boyle's law 9
brainstem 25, 27
branching morphogenesis 34–5
breathing
  abdominal 5
  paradoxical 5
  thoracic 5
breathing control
  chemical mechanisms 24–5
  neural mechanisms 26–7
bronchi 2–3, 38
  arteries 3
  breath sounds 45
  buds 35
  circulation 29
  provocation tests 59
  thermoplasty 59
bronchiectasis 39, 76–7
bronchioles 2, 3
bronchiolitis obliterans 75
bronchoalveolar lavage (BAL) 69
bronchomotor tone 14
bronchopleural fistula (BPF) 79
bronchopulmonary
  dysplasia 37
  nodes 3
  segments 3, 35
bronchoscopy 49
bronchus-associated lymphoid tissue
  (BALT) 41
buffers 20–21
  curves 21
  line 23
bulk flow 11

pulmonary (*continued*)
    tuberculosis 84–5
    vascular resistance 63
    vasculitis 66–7
purse-lipped breathing 61
pyramidal tracts 26–7

quadratus lumborum 4–5

radon gas 89
rapid eye movement (REM)
    sleep 97
reciprocal inhibition 27
recombinant anti-IgE antibodies 59
rectus abdominis 5
recurrent pneumonia 81
regulatory T cells (TReg) 41
relative humidity 9
renal compensation 23
residual volume (RV) 6–7
respiratory
    acidosis 23
    alkalosis 23
    bronchioles 3
    compensation 23
    disease 23
    failure 54–5
    failure, acute 23
    failure, chronic 23
    gas exchange ratio 19
    muscles 4–5, 26
    rhythm 27
resting tidal volume 6–7
restrictive disease 13
restrictive ventilatory defects
    (RVDs) 47
retroambiguus nucleus 26
rheumatoid arthritis 66–7
rhonchi (expiratory wheezes) 15
rhythm of respiration 27
ribs 4–5
right bronchi 3
right crus 4
right lung 3
right ventricular dysfunction 63
right-to-left shunts 28–9, 55

salbutamol 58–9, 61
salmeterol 58–9
sarcoidosis 70–71
saturated water vapour pressure 9
scalene muscles 5
scleroderma 66–7
SCUBA diving 33
segmental bronchi 3, 35
sensors 27
serratus anterior 5
sheath cells 25
shunt effect 31
silent zone 15
silicosis 75
silicotic nodules 75

skin prick tests 59
sleep apnoea 96–7
slow adaptation 27
small cell (SC) cancers 89
smoking 45, 52–3
    and asthma 57
    and lung cancer 89
smoking-related diseases
    (SRDs) 52
social factors 53
sodium cromoglycate 59
sol phase 39
spiral/helical computed
    tomography 65
spirometer
    bellows 7
    electrospirometer 7
    simple water-filled 7
splanchnic mesoderm 35
spontaneous ventilation (SV) 92
sputum pot 44
squamous cell cancers 89
squamous cell carcinomas 89
squamous epithelium 38
standard temperature and pressure dry
    (STPD) 9
Starling forces 29
static lung compliance 13
static pressure–volume (P–V) curve 12,
    13
sternal angle 2–3, 5
sternomastoids 5
sternum 4–5
stretch receptors 27
strong acids 21
structure of respiratory system 2–3
subcutaneous emphysema (SE) 79
submucosal glands 3, 39
sulphur dioxide 74
surface tension 12, 13
surfactant 3, 13, 35, 39
surfactant proteins 39
sympathetic trunk 3
synchronized intermittent mandatory
    ventilation (SIMV) 92–3
synergistic response 25
systemic capillary pressure 28
systemic circulation 29
systemic lupus erythematosus
    (SLE) 66–7

T cell receptors (TCRs) 41
tachypnoea 55, 65
tactile vocal fremitus 45
tank ventilator 93
taxol-based chemotherapy 89
terminal bronchioles 3
terminal sacs 35
tetralogy of Fallot 29
thalassaemia 37
Thebesian veins 28–9
theophylline 58–9

thermophilic actinomycetes 75
thoracic breathing 5
thoracic cage 3–5
thoracic vertebral column 5
thromboembolism 63–5
thrombolytics 65
tidal volume 6–7
time-derivative symbols 9
tiotropium 61
tissue hypoxia 95
tolerance 59
total lung capacity (TLC) 6–7
trachea 2–3, 38
    atresia 37
    stenosis 37
tracheobronchomegaly 36
tracheoesophageal fistula 37
transdiaphragmatic pressure 47
transoesophageal echocardiography 65
transudative pleural diseases 72–3
transverse fissures 3
travel history 45
true ribs 5
tubercle 5
tuberculosis (TB), pulmonary 84–5
tuberculous pleurisy 73
turbulent flow 14–15
type I alveolar pneumocytes 3, 11,
    38–9
type II alveolar pneumocytes 3, 11, 13,
    35, 38–9
type 1 respiratory failure 55
type 2 respiratory failure 55

uncontrolled asthma 59
unfractionated heparin (UFH) 65
upper respiratory tract 3
Urbach–Wiethe syndrome 36
usual interstitial pneumonitis (UIP/IPF)
    68–9

vagi 3
vagus nerve 24
varenicline 53
venae cordis minimae (VCM) 28–9
venous admixture 31
venous thromboembolism 64–5
ventilation–perfusion (V/Q)
    mismatch 30–31, 55
ventilation–perfusion (V/Q)
    scans 49
ventilator-associated pneumonia
    (VAP) 83
ventilator-induced lung
    damage 90
ventral respiratory group 26–7
vertebrochondral ribs 5
vertebrosternal ribs 5
vesicular breath sounds 45
viral infections and asthma 57
visceral pleura 3, 7
vital capacity 6–7